MW00638981

Anna Ghizzani

HEALTHY AGING:

Well-Being and Sexuality at Menopause and Beyond

novum pro

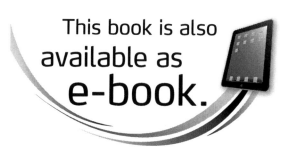

www.novumpublishing.com

© 2020 novum publishing

ISBN 978-1-64268-145-1
Editing: Karen Simmering
Cover photos: Brainsil,
Ihor Svetiukha | Dreamstime.com
Cover design, layout & typesetting:
novum publishing

www.novumpublishing.com

Contents

Introduction

Why this book?

I have been a gynecologist for almost forty years, and in my professional career I have had occasion to speak with many women about their health; as one may imagine, menopause has often been a major subject of these conversations. Over the years, I have found myself dealing more and more with this subject, partly because my patients and I simply happen to have grown older together, and partly because this biological process of menopause combines hormonal (endocrine) aspects with aspects to do with emotions and relationships, which I deal with as part of my second professional identity, as a qualified sexologist and sex therapist.

So I was the last person likely to be indifferent to the changes that the aging process brings about in a couple's sex life!

The unmistakable sign of menopause is the cessation of menstruation, caused by metabolic phenomena affecting the body (biological aspects) and one's emotions (psycological aspects), and it is accompanied by aging processes that follow independent biological mechanisms. Together, they are responsible for all those changes occurring in maturity that are not exactly "welcome." The way a person behaves, accepting these rather unwanted events, and taking the best from them, represents the key to aging in a positive way, while a slight vein of anxiety, or depression, is the mirror of one's reaction as one adjusts to the new situation.

In any transition phase, when life inevitably leads towards something that has to happen, and that may not always be pleasant, one needs a safe environment in which to voice one's doubts and – why not? – also one's fears. Generally, women do not seem to have a clear idea of what to expect in this phase of life, perhaps because the experience has not been passed on from one generation to the next; might it be possible that mothers have not wanted to worry their daughters prior to the event? This is likely. In any event, many women are in the dark as regards what lies beyond menstrual irregularities, and unfortunately they are also the target of information in the media which, by its popular nature, cannot be exhaustive, and cannot respond to the doubts of an individual person.

Many women express the need to know whether what they are going through is normal, what the limits of this normality are, how to combat a normality that worsens the quality of life, and especially how it is possible to realize whether a symptom is being transformed into an illness. Others ask whether the right thing to do is to treat minor complaints, with the certainty that medication will not cause worse damage. If we remember the controversy over hormone treatment for menopause that sprang up more than 10 years ago, and that has not yet been completely resolved, the dilemma is not as off-the-wall as it may seem. In this connection, I recall a former schoolfriend of mine, just over 40 at the time, who came to see me at the first symptoms of menopause. I spoke to her as delicately as I could about possible hormone therapy. In response, she showed me a page from a fashion magazine, and told me flatly that that regime was the cause of breast tumors, and was therefore to be rejected outright. By contrast, another friend regarded menopause as the most wonderful time of life for her, because it coincided with falling in love and marrying for the second time. Her happiness over her personal situation meant that she did not even notice the physical inconveniences!

A gynecologist is that doctor who is always sought when a patient has a complaint involving the genitals, or one of the functions exercised by that part of the body: reproduction/contraception, the urinary tract, and the sexual function. As such, a variety of requests are made to gynaecologists, but not all of these fall within her or his field of expertise. As a result, the gynecologist acquires considerable experience and knowledge of these requests, as well as women's expectations and their difficulties.

I feel particularly caught up in this mechanism, because, in my dual specialty of gynecologist and doctor of sexual medicine, I also treat men, and I have learnt to understand their emotions and their expectations regarding sexual health and relationships. I thus have the privilege of noting the joys and tribulations of the human spirit from a dual perspective.

After many years, I am still enthusiastic about my work, which I find highly interesting, creative, and always new. From the hours I have spent with my female patients came the idea for this book, that offers an overview of the issues associated with the two faces of the menopause: the normal (physiological) face, that only requires awareness and a little patience, and the more problematic face, for which medical intervention may be necessary.

I thank all of my patients for the trust they have shown me, and for having taught me the ability to listen, without which no diagnosis is possible, and no suitable intervention can be devised. Accordingly, this book is dedicated to them, and to whoever wants to get to know the myriad aspects of menopause as a physiological phenomenon, albeit a rather challenging one.

The issue of aging is more important now than in the past, given that the average lifespan has gotten longer. I believe that addressing menopause in a positive way, understanding its mechanisms and taking action against its negative effects, or, better still, preventing those negative effects, can be a wonderful way to tackle aging with determination: vitality, awareness, emotional balance and good health are the best ingredients for a journey that is set to remain a long one.

This volume is written in a good-natured way, to help women to understand somewhat better an event which affects them closely, in the hope that they may get useful infromation from it, as well as personal benefit. It is written also for those who, working in the health profession as care workers and therapists, want a few extra pointers for advising their patients as well as possible.

CHAPTER 1

What is Menopause?

An overview

Only recently has menopause become a subject of interest in itself, also to researchers. However, this should be no surprise. Indeed, at the start of the 20th century women in Europe had a life expectancy of just 48 years. This has gradually increased, thanks to progressive improvements in social and economic conditions in European countries. Today, unless one has a major metabolic disease, the average lifespan is 80 years; it is predicted that, in 2020, in the United States alone, there will be 46 million women over the age of 50 who could live another thirty years or so, namely a third of their lives, in menopause; according to UN projections, this figure is set to rise. In the year 2050, women aged 60 or over will make up 40% of the female population in Europe, and 23% of the global population, thanks to better and better living conditions. It is clear that in the Western world an ever higher number of older seniors, men and women, who have surpassed the age of 85, will maintain their intellectual vivacity, the product of a wellbeing that is more than just the absence of illness. By comparison, at the end of the second millennium, life expectancy in sub-Saharan Africa was just 52, and in many African nations it actually fell by three years, owing to the AIDS epidemic.

In the Western world, the average age of menopause is 51 or 52, a figure that has remained unchanged in the last few decades. However, the age is lower in women who have a poor socio-economic level.

Menopause as a biological phenomenon remains the same, but as a subjective experience it is today very different from the past, thanks to the fact that living conditions in Western countries have greatly improved compared to the early 1900s. Continual social progress affords us a level of wellbeing never seen before, with good quality food, comfortable housing, and the possibility of accessing increasingly effective medical care. The peak of sophistication in the medical field, the miracle which tends to go unnoticed, is the possibility of early diagnosis and, in some cases, even prevention. This is not the best of all possible worlds, as I am well aware, but the well-being that Western society has achieved was unthinkable up until just a few decades ago.

The first manifestations of menopause (usually a major delay in the cycle, or a series of hot flashes) always arrive unexpectedly. I don't know a single woman who has not said, somewhat agitatedly: "No, it's not possible, it's too soon! Doctor, what can it be?"

Many of these women, namely today's 50-somethings, are in an active phase of their lives, or even "super-active", because neither their working life nor their role in looking after the family has come to an end. There was a time when it was said that the years of menopause were emotionally difficult because they coincided with other important changes: children leaving home and leaving the world of work; there was talk of the "empty nest syndrome" to describe a family and social situation in which, after having been busy at home and outside the home for years, the woman found herself "unemployed." After a life spent juggling two full-time jobs, it suddenly seemed that nobody needed her any more, and it was supposed that this sense of not being needed might explain the mood swings and dissatisfaction that many women complained of. Today we are seeing that the social situation is completely different (the exact opposite of the "empty nest"!), because reproductive trends have changed, and many women have their first child around the age of 40. The life cycle remains the same, but the phases that comprise it have become longer: one enters the world of the workplace, and one thinks about a family later; of course, a woman in her 40s today no longer resembles the 40-somethings of 20 years ago, and, in terms of her life phases, this is the right time to think about a child.

Because one enters the world of work, and only thinks about starting a family at an older age, the nest of a woman who has just entered menopause, and who had a pregnancy around the age of 40, is populated by one or more lively adolescents who keep their mum constantly on the go.

In this respect, I see menopause as a new territory, whose essence is social rather than medical. Indeed, women in their 50s and 60s are the ones who have shown how many wonderful and gratifying things the years of one's "young old age" might still offer. They are women who, in growing older, have continued to remain naturally attractive, to work with creativity, to make room for interests that they were unable to pursue in their years of full-time employment, and who have enriched their emotional life by looking after grandchildren and the extended family. Credit for this lies not just with them; it also lies in the social development in which they have been fortunate enough to live, and to grow old. I can't help thinking that what we today regard as "normality" has been achieved thanks to the generations of women who, together with their men, paved the way for these privileges to become real.

Women entering menopause today belong to the generation of *Baby Boomers*, born in the prosperity of the post-war years, for whom parity of rights between the sexes and widespread access to education have been acquired rights to be fought for. Thus, the *Baby Boomers* were the trailblazers for the generations that followed, and they very much continue to be pioneers in this phase of their life, too. Arriving at menopause after having been privileged by culture and social well-being, this generation has basically established new models of behavior also in the medical field, because it was the first to become aware of the importance of replacement therapy, of prevention, and of early diagnosis of illnesses such as cancer of the uterus and breast cancer, as well as the first to decide to maintain professional and personal interests, and to choose an active lifestyle that fulfilled the biological needs of the elderly.

Kandinskij gives a wonderful image of the person who is the first to bring about a change, and describes this person as the tip of the iceberg, one that, on emerging, pulls along all the rest, who are still underwater. Similarly, women going through menopause today are paving the way for new behavioral models, and show how growing old today is an adventure that is yet to be written, owing to the infinite possibilities we have for maintaining a state of extended physical and emotional well-being, and also for attenuating its more disagreeable physical aspects.

Naturally, there are patients who present with purely medical ailments, such as uterine fibroids and heavy menstrual bleeding, and the problems of older women who have been problem-free in the initial phases, but, in the longer term, have developed ailments mainly linked to tissue atrophy. A less numerous group, but one no less important, comes to talk about sexuality, which has started to become problematic: sometimes because there is a loss of desire, sometimes owing to a physical difficulty, and other times owing to a difficulty on the part of their husband.

But why is it so important to get ready and enjoy life in the post-menopause years? The answer's simple! If menopause occurs shortly after turning 50, and women are living into their 80s on average, it follows that we will have more years to live after menopause than the whole duration of fertility. What's more, even the most glamorous 50-somethings eventually hit menopause: All women experience alterations of sleeping patterns, mood swings, changes in circulation (the notorious hot flashes!), and vaginal function (dryness that makes sexual relations difficult). While these are inevitable, one way or another – just like wrinkles! – they can, however, be considerably reduced in their seriousness by careful prevention.

We know that growing older is inevitable, and that one day we will be forced to reckon with a string of physical and mental limitations, but we also know that many resources are available in the West to enjoy life to the full, even in this phase of life. Qualitative improvements in lifestyle, and modern medical tools, afford opportunities that were previously unthinkable, and so looking backward at our grandmothers and mothers shaking their heads and refusing help, because "as they managed, so we will manage, too", is not the right attitude. Previous generations had a life expectancy that was around 10 years less than ours, and, for this simple reason, they were less exposed to the functional limitations of a debilitating and progressive illness such as osteoporosis and bone deformations. Certainly, to get results in the field of prevention it's not enough for the patient to have theoretical information: consultation with a doctor is needed to help people achieve this awareness.

Debunking myths and legitimate expectations

The task of a woman in her 50s is not to stay young forever; it's to build a future for herself in which her previous life represents her inheritance, and her future life represents opportunity. The future depends on expectations that a person has, and in some sense on their dreams.

The most absurd myth, or counter-myth, that needs to be debunked right from the start is that good looks don't matter! Anyone who says this is a liar, and a shameless liar. Good looks are important in every aspect of life, including the professional aspect. But while the beauty of adolescent models with perfect make-up who we admire in fashion magazines is beyond reach, the personal style of a real, fulfilled woman, who is happy with the way she is, and who takes good care of herself, is unbeatable. What does it mean to take good care of oneself? Well, it certainly consists in looking after one's physical well-being, which comes from exercise and a healthy diet. There is a wide choice of ways to maintain muscle tone and burn off a few calories along the way: one could go back to practicing a sport played in one's youth, which one perhaps was later forced to drop, or else try a completely new exercise with gentle physical activity that does not involve any danger of injury. These include yoga, Nordic walking and acquagym, or one could even simply start the habit of going to work on foot, or parking the car a few blocks further away. Actually, three or four hours a week of brisk walking are enough to lend our metabolism a hand, so… no excuses!

As regards diet, the same applies, to some extent: There is no need for heroism (what would the world be like without Nutella?); a little commonsense is all it takes. Just organize your meals so you can relax and enjoy them with friends and family, and make sure that your lunch break is actually a real break from work, possibly with one or two co-workers (why not?). A moment of socialization improves one's mood and helps to keep the amount of food under control.

After all, healthy eating in Italy is easy; for years our diet has been recognized as the most balanced, including seasonal products rich in fibers, vitamins and salts that are cooked without too many fats. Of course, there is no such thing as a miracle menu (the most popular are based on boiled fish and fresh vegetables) but, apart from the dominant factor of genetic predisposition, a healthy diet has the most important role in safeguarding health. The benefits are seen in a lower incidence of diabetes, hypertension and cardiocirculatory disease, and that is why it is absolutely necessary to be careful and aware.

The human body is a collection of organs that work in close contact with each other, and it is inconceivable that the health (or otherwise) of each does not influence the next. This goes beyond the physiological aspect, and also includes the domain of feelings and emotions, in which there are many more variables.

Well-being is often also down to interpersonal relations, built up over the years. This gives rise to a way of living that includes a range of attachments, such as old and new friends, pastimes and interests that help to develop a network of social relations, and obviously the family ties that time consolidates, smoothes, and makes more mellow.

While we're at it, let's debunk another stereotype: women of a certain age no longer progress in their careers… Says who? With the benefit of her accumulated experience and self-assurance, a motivated woman can achieve any goal without needing to compete against younger women, or she can also decide to make a radical new departure in her working life. In this, women are freer than men, partly because by nature they are more aware of their needs, and partly because society puts them under less pressure. A woman aged 50, the age when menopause reigns supreme, can freely choose to dedicate her time to more gratifying activities, and not consider the deadlock in her career as a failure: there are one's loved ones, her long-term companion and her personal interests, from which up until now she has stolen time. Are we certain that this decision is less commendable?

Occurrence and variability of the menstrual cycle

The cessation of menstrual cycles signals the moment that for every woman represents the beginning of menopause and of the endocrine phemomena that characterize aging. Plasma levels of follicle-stimulating hormone (FSH) and luteinizing hormone (LH) begin to increase a few years before the end of menstruations, as concentrations of estradiol and progesterone gradually fall, proving that the ovary becomes gradually less responsive to the action of gonadotrophins; in this phase, cycles may maintain a regular pattern for a lengthy period of time, but they become anovulatory.

It is thought that decreased ovarian responsiveness to gonadotropins (regulators of hormonal production) is the trigger of menopause, and that most of its characteristic symptoms are the effect of the ensuing lower production of estrogen. The symptom resulting from these biochemical phenomena is a significant menstrual irregularity: periods can disappear suddenly and permanently, or return for an unpredictable number of months, and have variable characteristics; they may become lighter and less frequent, become completely irregular, or maintain a regular rhythm with minimal blood loss, or else involve heavy bleeding.

Other typical menopausal signs that affect every woman are vasomotor instability, atrophic involution of the organs that are targets of estrogen stimulation (the breasts, external genitals, and womb), and mood changes. Vasomotor instability causes hot flashes, sudden hot sensations in the face and neck, with redness of skin and profuse sweating, while genital atrophy involves the thinning of the vulvar plicae and of the vaginal mucosa, which lowers resistance to microorganisms, and makes sexual intercourse difficult.

The direct impact of menopause on these symptoms is clear; by contrast, it is difficult to define its relationship with a number of symptoms concerning emotions: nervousness, anxiety, a depressive attitude, and sleep disturbances, bringing about mood changes that, in turn, reduce general well-being, increase fatigue, make it difficult to concentrate, and lower the energy to perform everyday tasks; but, like genital atrophy, they may also have a negative influence on relationships, and interfere with sexual desire and sexual gratification.

How does menopause occur?

The long process of physiological (ie normal) menopause begins with an initial phase called perimenopause; this is the period characterized by the fact the ovarian function gradually becomes irregular, with decreasing estrogen production. The entire organism reacts to the changing hormonal environment with vasomotor symptoms (hot flashes), disruption of sleep architecture (insomnia and waking up too early), and mood disturbances (a tendency to be anxious). Perimenopause, or menopausal transition, may last for a couple of years, until depletion of the reproductive capability. During this period the menstrual rhythm becomes extremely variable.

Quite common symptoms are difficulty in falling asleep, a tendency towards anxiety and depression and crying without reason, irritability and difficulty in concentrating on things one has to do, some memory deterioration, and frequent headaches that were not present at an earlier age. Other symptons, such as a tingling feeling, night sweats, and the need to urinate frequently, are not so frequent. During the menopausal transition this set of symptoms, in various combinations, is present to a moderate degree, and in transient form, in at least 2 women out of every 3, while in about 10% of patients it continues for some years, in some cases in a severe fashion, and in others to a gradually lesser degree over time.

In some cases, it may happen that mild symptoms worsen as time goes by, but most often they start out as severe in the first year, and then trail off. It seems that the sense of well-being and the ability to keep symptoms under control increase in women with a higher level of education, and that women who are in a fulfilling relationship are able to put up with the disturbances more easily. It is likely that this represents a positive response to feeling understood and emotionally supported.

Finally, at some point menstruations cease altogether, either naturally or with pharmacological help. The symptoms that marked perimenopause may lessen, disappear, or remain present during the phase called stabilized menopause, while other symptoms (regarded as presenting later than usual) gradually become evident as the years go by. These are osteoporosis and atrophy of the genitourinary tract. These are normal symptoms, but only within certain limits; if their clinical characteristics become more severe, full-scale illnesses develop, requiring specific medical intervention; this is why it is important for patients to be able to recognize when a discomfort turns into an actual ailment.

In specific conditions, transition and stabilization of menopause take place in different forms.

Premature menopause

This term describes the demise of the cycle in women below the age of 40. The condition, called premature ovarian insufficiency (POI), affects about 1% of the population. As such, it is relatively frequent, and represents a devastating life experience for young women affected by it. For the sake of completeness, it should be mentioned that the condition may not be 100% stable, unlike the natural menopause; indeed, there have been pregnancies, although very rarely, in patients diagnosed with POI.

The dysfunction is caused by an ovarian defect that depletes the follicles long before the physiological time, leading to infertility, a condition that today has a more serious social impact than in the past, as the tendency is to have children later in their lives. A young woman who develops ovarian insufficiency after having already had children will have to deal with a major metabolic imbalance, but, in the event of her losing her reproductive capability, she will also face psychological symptoms.

It is not yet clear what causes ovarian insufficiency, but scientists recognize at least a concomitant genetic component. The empirical observation that daughters ressemble their mothers in many endocrine and reproductive aspects is backed up by sound scientific data.

A number of authors report that POI has been found in families of different ethnic backgrounds, such as Hispanics, Anglo-Saxons, Italians, and Ashkenazi Jews, where grandmothers, mothers, sisters, and cousins develop the same pattern of premature ovarian insufficiency more or less at the same age. Knowing that the ailment runs in families is vital for being able to advise women affected by this genetic risk factor how to best use their reproductive capabilities.

Despite the patient's young age, the cessation of the ovarian function causes infertility and the metabolic pattern of menopause, with a clinical impact that is accentuated by the fact that the symptoms appear suddenly and forcefully rather than gradually, as in natural menopause. If a patient has not yet accomplished her project for a family when she develops premature menopause, and would have wanted more children, the emotional impact of being forced to give up her plans can be utterly negative, and can change for the worse the patient's quality of life. Other justifiable concerns involve the long-term effects of estrogen deprivation. In particular, one concern is loss of calcium. The onset of this is triggered by low estrogen values many years before the normal physiological time, leading to osteoporosis; negative mood fluctuations in response to this unnatural condition, when present, constitute a pathology in itself, affecting one's general well-being.

Iatrogenic or induced menopause

This is the menopausal state caused before its natural time by medical interventions, which can be more or less invasive. The most frequent ones are the bilateral removal of the ovaries, treatment to suppress estrogen production, and radiation and chemotherapy, namely therapeutical regimes prescribed for diseases of extremely different severity.

As an example, let's consider a surgical procedure, hysterectomy, that is very common but does not indicate a severe pathology. Hysterectomy, meaning the surgical removal of the womb, may be recommended for mild conditions such as the presence of myomas, and it is performed with or without the simultaneous ablation of the ovaries. When the uterus is removed but not the ovaries, a woman does not have her cycle any more (meaning that she is menopausal by definition), and could not become pregnant, but she maintains a regular hormonal concentration that protects her from the aforementioned damage from premature menopause. Unfortunately, performing a hysterectomy while leaving the ovaries in place is not always possible, because the organs are very close to each other. In the past, this was not considered a problem because the general belief was that ovaries would lose their function once the reproductive phase had come to an end. Today we know that their endocrine activity continues throughout a woman's life, even though in reduced amounts; consequently their surgical removal without a specific justification is strongly discouraged.

Unfortunately, in the long term, even healthy ovaries left in place become dysfunctional and reduce their estrogen secretion within five years after hysterectomy, most likely because the surgical alteration suffered by the tissues damages the circulatory system, resulting in insufficient blood flow that makes the ovaries age before their time.

The suppression of estrogen production is recommended in endometriosis, a disease that presents itself during the reproductive years with diffuse pain in the lower pelvis, in coincidence with ovulation, menstrual cycles, sexual intercourse, and the passing of urine and feces. The disease is caused by the presence of endometrial material outside of the uterus, and the intensity of pain worsens during the menstrual phases characterized by higher estrogen concentration; therefore, their suppression is advisable in order to alleviate the symptoms.

What are the consequences of induced menopause for women suffering from this condition?

Everything hinges upon the secondary effects of estrogen loss, exactly as happens with the occurrence of premature menopause as described above; in this instance, too, the clinical pattern is made more severe compared to natural menopause, because production ends abruptly, not allowing the long period of adjustment that is part of the natural mechanisms.

Symptoms can only be alleviated within the limits determined by the condition that induced the menopause.

In the case of hysterectomy, we have a healthy patient whose ovaries have been removed because it was technically impossible to preserve them during surgery. In this instance, we are free to choose any treatment regime that seems the most suitable. On the other hand, we know that the suppression of estrogen in the bloodstream is vital to reduce the symptoms of endometriosis. Therefore, in this case, our arsenal of treatments must be limited to medications that do not contain hormones, or to local use of these.

A separate category comprises young women who are not yet menopausal, and who develop a tumor that is responsive to estrogen. This pathology requires a medication capable of suppressing estrogen production, and that is prescribed in addition to surgical ablation and radiation therapy to enhance their effectiveness. Its role is to block the production of estrogens "feeding" the tumor. Inevitably, therefore, side effects will occur such as irregular or absent cycles, vasomotor symptoms, and vaginal atrophy. In addition, a decrease has been reported in sexual desire, but in my opinion this should not be considered separately from the emotional impact that a potentially deadly condition has on a patient's psychological equilibrium.

An oncology patient must take strong medication, leading to damaging side effects that most often cannot be avoided. It is encouraging to know that a menopause-like symptom, namely vulvo-vaginal atrophy, can be cautiously treated with specific sexual medicine interventions, possibly leading to an improvement.

Cycles of life

When one talks about menopause, one sometimes has in mind the image of a woman who has already left the world of work, because up until relatively recently it was possible for the two things to coincide. Now the rules have changed, and the two events arrive a few years apart from each other. This period can make a difference in a person's psychophysical state; but above all one must bear in mind that they occur in response to two very differing mechanisms, one biological and the other social. In any event, it is understandable that they should be associated with each other in discussions of this time of life, because the two phenomena, although very distinct from each other, also resemble each other. Indeed, both mark the end of one era (one's working life and fertile life), and the beginning of another.

Menopause at 50

The metabolic processes of aging present very gradually, allowing people to grow accustomed to wrinkles, having to wear glasses, slowing down, and so on. The onset of menopause speeds up these small inconveniences and brings new ones with it, ones resulting more directly from hormonal changes: more fatigue and less concentration, a sense of general malaise, and the beginning of a number of sexual difficulties make daily life less easy, and are slightly humiliating. The way a woman perceives this experience depends on cultural acceptance of the slow, treacherous, irreversible and inevitable changes that occur in older people, because being comfortable with oneself comes from an awareness of being appreciated. A positive approach makes it easier to maintain a healthy lifestyle, and the motivation to look after oneself, involving the use of available medical and social resources, such as the services of preventive medicine, and places where one can meet others socially. In other words, it means maintaining the ability to make decisions for oneself.

Leaving the world of work

Around the age of 60, people are called "young old people" in order to underline the fact that, alongside one's self-evident maturity, one also finds the opportunities of a free age, if not exactly a second youth, during which many favorable aspects can be enjoyed. Leaving the world of work gives one hours and hours of personal freedom; but this is not the only option, because one could choose to reduce the amount of work one does without abandoning work altogether. In this way, one would have a dual opportunity to maintain an interest and have more flexibility.

The conditions for enjoying these years to the full are being in good health and having special people with whom one can share one's plans. A loving relationship, a close-knit family, and a group of friends are vital for exploring the world. Those who, for whatever reason, find themselves alone see their chances of establishing a position in society reduced, because it is discouraging to take initiatives without anyone to share them with. Whereas in previous times a certain kind of social solitude could be countered by having a job and its associated activities, this opportunity is now no longer present after retirement. As one gets older, arriving at menopause, and in the run-up to quitting the world of the workplace, emotional solitude becomes more keenly felt, especially if the result of a divorce, or being widowed, the two life events that are regarded as those that are hardest to deal with psychologically. After age 50, it becomes less and less likely that people who are potentially compatible and equally desirous of a romantic relationship get to meet each other. Finding oneself without a romantic relationship that fulfills one's need for intimacy and sharing is a situation that affects both men and women. By contrast, it has been shown that solitude represents the biggest threat to psychophysical well-being. In a social context such as that of the West, where it is relatively common for couples to divorce, it is clear that people living alone desire a relationship even when they are older. Thus, despite the difficulty in meeting the right person, second marriages and cohabitation are ways of allowing people to find new gratification, joy and emotional stability.

Single women

A situation of social difficulty that is hard to resolve affects women who are left alone after being widowed, or because of a relationship break-up. This affects a higher number of women than men, because women benefit most from increased life expectancy. Older people who do not have specific illnesses find themselves in a state of physical and mental health that allows them to remain active in their profession and creative in their personal life. Alongside intellectual vivacity, very much present is the desire for a fulfilling relationship that offers intimacy and sharing. In a social context such as life in the West, where it is common for couples to divorce, it is logical that many single women should wish to start a new relationship even in their older years in order to find new gratification, joy and emotional stability. Unfortunately, however, it is hard for a mature woman to meet a suitable male partner who is interesting, and who shows himself to be interested, even though men left by themselves as a result of the vicissitudes of life seem to desire a relationship as much as women do. Basically, opportunities for people with these characteristics to meet are rare, especially in small towns; this unfortunate fact seriously interferes with an aspiration that is more than legitimate, and contributes in maintaining a state of solitude, which is the biggest threat to psychophysical well-being.

The difficulties in forming a new relationship seem to be especially social in nature, insofar as people with a well-constructed life behind them, and with family relations and friendships that have a very important emotional role, may not manage to combine a life of emotional attachments with a "new arrival" who might upset the previous equilibrium. Living in distant towns and cities, having very differing lifestyles, but especially maintaining family commitments, or work-related or social commitments that are incompatible with the availability that a new life requires are obstacles to the formation of a new couple. The attitude of society, which, still today, is not always open to the sexuality of older people, could create difficulty for a person who is perhaps particularly sensitive to the approval of others, and who undertakes an active search for a new partner. It is nevertheless true that social norms are always evolving, and are becoming gradually less restrictive, allowing a greater fluidity in forming a new relationship in every kind of circumstance. Equally, a positive view of relationships between older people is certainly more widespread than before, perhaps also because, with the rise in divorces, there is a more widespread need by many people to form a new family.

As often happens in many other aspects of life, people who are more strong-willed and determined to fulfill their needs dare to embark upon changes and are often rewarded. Let's not forget that today's 60-somethings were the original *Baby Boomers*, the generation that marked a break, the generation of post-war prosperity, rebellion, and the search for freedom of expression. The rebellious stance, sometimes taken to extremes, that has always been one of their characteristics, now proves to be very useful in facilitating a more open attitude towards new meetings. Since they were also the first generation that, right from the start of their sexual lives, had access to a range of safe methods of contraception that were easy to use and readily available, they have always been used to regarding sex as a valuable aspect in the life of an individual, and in the life of a couple, distinct from the reproductive function. They are certainly aware that problems increase with age: now sex is more fragile, and cannot be taken for granted. However, this does not become an impediment to the search for a relationship, and indeed the findings of many research studies, despite the fact they do not wholly agree with each other, seem to suggest that menopause, with all its range of associated symptoms that are not always pleasant, does not necessarily have to change emotional intimacy and fulfillment.

One birthday after another, with a smile!

During the whole period of writing this book, my mind was focused on women between the ages of 50 and 70, perhaps influenced by the fact that most patients fall into this age bracket, and it is in these years that they need to be accompanied in order to move from transition to stabilized menopause.

This is an understandable clinical approach, and it has a certain *raison d'etre*. However, if I look around, in the street, at the cinema or at the hairdresser's, my construction proves to be insufficient, because it neglects other women, the ones over the age of 70, who are just as interesting, active and in control of their own lives, and they deserve to be taken into account. These ladies, however, have a different biological make-up, and so they require specific attention.

On average, women in their 70s have been in a state of stabilized menopause for more than 10 years, and so they do not need interventions to guide them through the adjustment period. Indeed, for these patients there are contraindications in beginning a treatment based on ovarian hormones. Nevertheless, they can still do a lot to maintain, or improve, their quality of life.

Well-being is the product of a fit body and a positive mind. Having ensured freedom of movement means independence for daily needs, and the possibility of maintaining recreational activities and friendships, while a positive psychological attitude means valuing oneself and one's life.

Although they influence each other, these two conditions are independent of each other. For the former, all the physical activity that one's health allows is recommended. Whether it is light exercise, aquagym, yoga or walking… everything helps to maintain agility, slow down the process of osteoporosis, and also enjoy a few more occasions for socialization. It has been proven that a well-devised program of regular physical exercise improves cognitive functions, as well as one's mood, and that maintaining interests and social relations offers emotional fulfillment that helps one to age well.

Among women over the age of 70, many no longer have an interest in sex, especially if they suffer from pelvic conditions, genital atrophy, or depression, but more women than is believed maintain a sex life. In most cases, these are close couples who have been able to adapt to the pathologies of aging in order to maintain intimacy even in non-perfect conditions, and who say that they are very satisfied with their decision, that makes it possible to maintain an intimate and lively relationship.

What's more, around 20% of women and men over the age of 80 have an active sex life, even though desire, frequency and the ability to be aroused are diminished[1]. The sexual activity of people over the age of 80 includes mutual masturbation, and, more rarely, intercourse[2].

Also at a less advanced age there are very real difficulties affecting both men and women that doctors can treat. In older women, genital atrophy interferes, inevitably and seriously, with maintaining an active sex life. This condition responds well to targeted, new-generation medicines, especially when it is associated with specific interventions involving sexual and behavioral therapy.

Further reading:

Treloar A. E., *Menstrual cyclicity and the pre-menopause* in «Maturitas», Elsevier, Amsterdam, 1981, pp. 249–264.

Greendale G. A, Sowers M., Han W., et al. *Bone mineral density loss in relation to the final menstrual period in a multiethnic cohort: Results from the Study of Women's Health Across the Nation* in "J Bone Miner Res", Wiley, Hoboken, 2012, pp. 111–118.

Neer R.M, *Bone loss across the menopausal transition*, in "Annals of the New York Academy of Science", Wiley, Hoboken, 2010, pp. 66–71.

Kalantaridou S.N., Nelson L.M., *Premature ovarian failure is not premature menopause,* in "Annals of the New York Academy of Science", Wiley, Hoboken, 2000, pp. 393–402.

---

1 Lee, Nazroo, O'Connor *et alii, Sexual health and well-being among older men and women in England: Findings from the English Longitudinal Study of Ageing,* in "Arch. Sex Behav.", vol. 45, 2016, pp.133–144.

2 Smith, Mulhall, Deveci *et alii Sex after seventy: A pilot study of sexual function in older persons,* in "J. Sex. Med.", vol. 4, 2007, pp. 1247–1253.

Mattison D.R., Evans M.I., Schwimmer W.B. *et al.*, *Familial Premature Ovarian Failure* in "The American Journal of Human Genetics", Elsevier, Amsterdam, 1984, pp. 1341–1348,

Rossetti R., Ferrari I., Bonomi M., Persani L., *Genetics of primary ovarian insufficiency* in "Clinical Genetics", Wiley, Hoboken, 2017, pp. 183–198.

CHAPTER 2

Medical Aspects:
Symptoms and Effects in Women

Vasomotor symptoms

Hot flashes, or flushing, are vasomotor symptoms that appear as an immediate response to a reduced level of estrogen in the blood-stream; since this reduction precedes the onset of the changes brought by the menstrual cycle, one or two isolated flashes may occur even when the cycle is still apparently regular. The intensity and frequency vary from woman to woman: for some, they are little more than an annoyance, while for others they represent a real problem, owing to the feelings of awkwardness that come with them. We should not overlook the effects of a hot flash when it comes "in public", because the redness and sweating are embarrassing, and make evident a situation that one would prefer to keep private. When these occur in the middle of a working day, they limit the ability to concentrate, make one feel inadequate, produce anxiety, and end up interfering in one's professional life and social relations. It seems that greater acceptance of hot flashes is associated with a positive mental outlook, good family relations, and general emotional well-being. They manifest with brief and sudden episodes of intense heat, located especially in the torso, the neck and the face, accompanied by redness and profuse sweating.

Their occurrence is extremely varied; they may represent a fleeting phenomenon, or begin before changes in the cycle, and remain for many years. When symptoms are severe, it becomes necessary to intervene with medication, to lessen the frequency and intensity of the episodes, so as to improve the patient's quality of social life, or else to allow them an adequate night's sleep – something not to be underestimated! Hot flashes are caused by the reduction in estrogen, but they present most frequently when a person is going through a stressful time.

However, findings from research studies observing patients from various different ethnic groups present us with differing realities. The symptoms of Chinese women are mainly tiredness, muscular pains, irritability, sleep disturbances, and muscular pains, which are also common among Japanese women, who, in turn, complain of memory loss and stress, but do not have hot flashes, instead reporting episodes of cold, which are another aspect of menopausal vasomotor instability. The incidence of hot flashes seems completely different in South American women; indeed, more than half report serious or very serious vasomotor symptoms. Other studies confirm that only 10–20% of Filippino women have hot flashes or episodes of night sweats, unlike 60–90% of women in Europe and the US. Initial observation suggests that ethnic variations cannot easily be explained, even if one takes into account high soya consumption among Asian women, as a protective factor.

What do patients ask for?

Requests for help for vasomotor symptoms (so difficult to accept) are very common in a gynecology clinic. Before resorting to medicine, it is right and proper for the patient to try to alleviate them with a lifestyle that pays attention to clothing, the environment, and nutrition. General advice valid for all women includes dressing in layers, so as to avoid feeling hot, lowering the temperature in the rooms where one lives, especially in the bedroom, getting mild but constant exercise, and avoiding spicy foods, wine, and cigarettes. It is important to maintain a suitable body weight, because overweight women are those who suffer most from these disturbances.

Women who cannot resolve the problem often look to nutritional supplements for a solution. These include soya isoflavones and red clover, which have a bland estrogen action, while cimicifuga (actaea) racemosa (black cohosh) is a serotonin agonist, a substance that regulates the response of the nervous system.

Low doses of new-generation antidepressants seem to work better than soya derivatives, but they can have unpleasant secondary effects on sexual behavior, because they slow down orgasm, and so they must be chosen on the basis of individual needs and preferences.

Naturally, hormone replacement therapy (HRT), which we will discuss later on, represents the most effective intervention, but a family history of breast cancer and risk factors for cardiocirculatory diseases mean there are contraindications over its use, and it is right that a patient should try possible alternative solutions before resorting to hormonal preparations.

Even though vasomotor symptoms do not harm the organism, they are truly irritating. However, the discomfort ultimately proves to be a welcome event, because it leads women to their doctor, giving them the opportunity to get advice about the real conditions, such as genital atrophy or osteoporosis, which must be tackled with preventive measures.

Cardiovascular diseases

Cardiovascular pathologies, and in particular coronary disease, are the most frequent cause of death in women. The pathological mechanism is similar to that in men, but with a number of characteristics specific to the female gender, depending on the amount of estrogen[3] in circulation, the reduction in which represents an important risk factor. This information is not taken on board by the public at large, and breast cancer, rather than cancer in any other organ, is the event most feared by middle-aged women. This fear is understandable if one thinks of the devastating impact that a cancer diagnosis has for a person, whatever organ is affected, and the special meaning that the breast has for any woman. However, it is not justified by the statistics. Indeed, a

---

3 Female sexual hormones produced by the ovarian follicles.

cardiovascular event is the most frequent cause of death in women (46% of cases), more than tumors, respiratory conditions, infectious diseases, cerebrovascular events and traumas. After the age of 50, causes of death in women are ischemic conditions, tumors, and neuromuscular degenerative diseases. Progress in the early diagnosis of tumors is improving the chances of survival, and increasing the incidence of ischemic conditions. Up until age 40, ischemic disease is less frequent in women, but after 50 it increases considerably, probably because with menopause one loses the protective effect of estrogen on the cardiovascular system.

The natural history of cardiac disease in women is different from that in men. Its first manifestation occurs with *angina pectoris* (chest pain caused by myocardial ischemia), instead of with a heart attack (65% and 35% respectively). The symptoms can remain less severe for years, and indeed women who suffer a heart attack are 7 or 8 years older than men.

After the age of 64, hypertension is the most frequent cause of cardiac stroke. Smoking is also an important risk factor in determining coronary disease and atherosclerosis in women without other health problems. Obesity, diabetes, and an altered lipid profile are factors that worsen damage caused by hypertension and smoking. Obesity by itself does not represent a direct risk for cardiovascular disease, but it does cause metabolic conditions such as hypercholesterolemia, and it worsens hypertension, events which have knock-on effects, contributing to coronary damage.

Oral contraceptives, such as the pill, only very rarely cause non-fatal heart attacks in women without other risk factors, but who are over the age of 40, or in younger women who are carriers of congenital heart disease, malign hypertension and cardiomyopathy. The most serious side effect caused by these drugs, is phlebothrombosis; for this reason, they are advised against in women with obesity and hypertension, or in women with an altered lipid profile[4].

---

4 Johansson-Vedin-Wilhelmsson, *Myocardial infarction in women* in "Epidemiologic Reviews", vol. 5, 1983, pp. 67–95.

The association between cigarette smoking and coronary ischemic damage is, however, well known. Around 30% of deaths from heart attacks can be ascribed to smoking, which is the biggest independent risk factor that can be changed, both for men and for women, and it correlates directly to the number of cigarettes smoked. Smoking two packets a day increases the risk by 200% compared to a non-smoker, and when smoking is associated with other factors, such as hypertension, the overall risk becomes greater than the mathematical sum of the two components. The risk of developing coronary disease and atherosclerosis (namely damage to blood vessels) remains significant in women who are smokers without other relevant factors, but in this case, too, the synergic relationship of smoking associated with taking oral contraceptives increases the risk of ischemic disease tenfold, compared to women who do not smoke, and who do not take contraceptives[5].

Differences between women and men

Cardiovascular disease is found to be the leading cause of death among women, despite the fact that it is extremely infrequent up until menopause. Ischemic damage, a heart attack, is between twice and four times as frequent in men than in women, but it is not clear what determines this difference; indeed, the higher incidence in men does not seem to be exclusively related to known risk factors (hypertension, body weight, diabetes, physical activity, and cholesterol levels). Indeed, if one looks at the problem from the point of view of the female gender, it seems that the low incidence of cardiocirculatory illness in pre-menopause ages can be put down to the protective effect that estrogen has on blood

---

5 Centers for Disease Control, *Smoking and cardiovascular disease*, in "MMWR", 1984, pp. 677–679.

vessel function. Other female characteristics include a lower propensity to develop hypercholesterolemia and diabetes, together with less stiffening of the peripheral arteries; this latter condition is to be ascribed to the direct action of estrogens on the vascular system, in which they cause arterial vasodilation and relaxation of the vascular muscles, with a resultant lowering of blood pressure. Together with their action to combat atherosclerosis, these constitute a powerful protective effect against hypertension.

The increased risk of cardiovascular disease in postmenopause may be due to hormonal changes and the aging process, although the relationship is not completely clear. In the same way, there is debate over the effect that replacement therapy in menopause has on the cardiocirculatory system, insofar as it has shown positive, negative and neutral effects in the course of many assessments. In any event, although the risk of cardiovascular disease in women increases with menopause, the greater susceptibility of men remains throughout their lives[6].

Cardiovascular conditions in menopause

Age is the factor of most importance for cardiovascular health, and women past the age of 50 see a great increase in their risk, although a direct relationship between the menopausal state and the beginning of the condition has never been detected; by contrast, an increased metabolic risk for cardiovascular conditions is recognised in the case of women who arrive at menopause with a diabetic or hypertensive condition.

Some findings suggest that there is a higher risk of thromboembolism if menopause sets in at an age above 52, or below 39,

---

6 Albrektsen, Heuch Løchen, Thelle, Wilsgaard, Njølstad, Bønaa, *Lifelong gender gap in risk of incident myocardial infarction: The Tromsø study* in "JAMA Internal Medicine", vol. 176, 2016, pp. 1673–1679.

while an age of between 40 and 49 at the time of the last menstrual cycle seems to constitute a protective factor.

During a woman's fertile years, estrogen acts on blood coagulation and on the function of arterial vessels, increasing the factors that facilitate coagulation, and reducing the factors that oppose it; furthermore, they promote dilation of the peripheral vessels, thereby helping to control blood pressure.

At menopause estrogen reduction and the mechanisms of aging alter this process. Aging influences the function of the arteries by means of the reduction of the vascular lumen, and the capacity to dilate in response to the estrogen stimulus. The loss of elasticity in the walls of the vessels is one component in the rise of blood pressure. The function of coronary arteries seems much better in young women than in men of the same age, and as much as twice as good as that in women in menopause, but differences are not found when one compares women in menopause with men of the same age.

Hormone therapy and the cardiovascular system

In view of the protective role played by estrogens during the years of fertility, it has been supposed that taking them in menopause might reduce cardiovascular risk.

It has been suggested that hormone replacement therapy might reduce mortality due to cardiovascular causes in postmenopausal women, and that it might have a beneficial effect on the lipid profile, on vasodilation, and on the integrity of the vascular wall, but the hoped-for benefit has not been confirmed. This is because estrogens given systemically increases the risk of thrombosis by acting on the activation of factors of coagulation, and on the greater production of thrombin. The use of estrogens taken through the skin (such as medicated patches) does not appear to be associated with an increase in haemostasis or coagulation, but neither does it offer benefits. Moreover, the scientific literature has not shown any positive effect from administering it with the aim of preventing or delaying a cardiovascular or cerebrovascular accident in women who have had episodes in the past. With the knowledge currently available, neither does it have benefits in the prevention of cardiovascular accidents in women without previous events[7].

Given that hormone replacement therapy does not have known benefits in preventing cardiovascular risk, it may be used in a patient who has entered menopause only recently to alleviate vasomotor symptoms, and for the prevention of osteoporosis, if there are no risks of cardiovascular or thromboembolic disease, or of breast cancer.

Osteoporosis

Osteoporosis means a weakening of the structure of bones, owing to the rarefaction of the medullary part, and, in my opinion, it is the most important issue to be addressed when a woman enters menopause. Let's remember that this syndrome is called "the silent killer", because it does not show itself until it is too late, at least as regards a treatment that has significant benefits, nor can it be prevented in advance. Unfortunately, manifestations of osteoporosis are always very harmful to a woman's health, with disabling fractures of the femur, the wrists, and the spinal column that are almost always caused by very slight traumas, or even spontaneous ones; the disease is responsible for a permanent state of pain in the spinal column, and the cause of bone deformations and bad posture. The damage is so serious because the loss of bone matrix is not evident, and there is no way to detect

---

7 Whayne, Mukherjee, *Women, the menopause, hormone replacement therapy and coronary heart disease* in "Curr Opin Cardiol", vol. 30, 2015, pp. 432–438.

it without carrying out a specific examination, a mineralometry, on a regular, repeated basis. If the problem goes unnoticed and is neglected, it is very likely that one will end up suffering from the aforementioned conditions.

What is the natural history of the absorption of calcium in bones? Calcium is absorbed from foods and fixed in bones by means of sunlight activating vitamin D in the skin. In optimum conditions, when exposure to sunlight, calcium intake, and estrogens in the bloodstream are sufficient, calcium is fixed to the bone matrix in large quantities up until the age of 20; it continues to be fixed more weakly up until age 30, and thereafter we see the opposite phenomenon: from the age of 30 onwards, calcium content in bones falls at a constant and slow rate until the onset of menopause. Estrogens have a second positive effect on bone metabolism, inasmuch as it maintains the power – ie the capacity for work – of muscle mass, which is a further factor that promotes calcium absorption.

When it comes to the functional limitations that a woman perceives as a sign of biological change, the first such involves the loss of muscle power, which in practical terms means that greater effort is needed to perform normal daily tasks; indeed, the extent to which muscle mass and strength are reduced determines how tiring tasks become that were once considered to be almost trivial. As well as diminishing the capacity for work, loss of muscle mass contributes to an associated loss of bone mass because it reduces the demands placed by muscles on the skeleton, which is a factor that encourages calcium absorption. The synergy between muscle work and maintaining bone mass is facilitated by testosterone, and represents one of the reasons why men fix more bone in their youth, and lose it less during aging, and are protected against osteoporosis. Unlike men, women start to lose muscle mass and strength around the age of 50, coinciding with menopause; the functional limitations described are accentuated as the years go by, with the biological phenomena of aging, and with the gradual reduction of steroids. Women who have had surgical menopause are those who suffer most from these phenomena because at the time of the removal of the ovaries, testosterone is suddenly reduced by 50%, making it hard for the biological systems to adapt to a change that, in natural menopause, occurs gradually over a period of many months.

Let's go back over some history: the cradle of mankind is in Africa, a land inundated with sun. Primitive man came into existence with particularly dark skin, which lets through the amount of sunlight necessary to activate the precursor of vitamin D, and at the same time protects against too much sun. Far back in time, man began to migrate towards northern lands, and dark skin represented an evolutionary disadvantage, because too much pigment did not allow the activation of vitamin D; without this, calcium is not fixed, and rickets sets in, with weak and deformed bones. The presence of a flat pelvis, which prevents a woman from giving birth, would have meant the extinction of the human race, had evolutionary mechanisms not determined an advantage in favour of people with pale skin, in which the low content of melanin does not block the sun's action on vitamin D.

In very northern regions, such as Canada, for six months of the year there is not enough sunlight to activate the forerunner of vitamin D, and to ensure good bone metabolism. The commonest foodstuffs, such as milk, have added vitamin D. But sun and vitamin D are not the only factors in bone metabolism. A significant role is also played by sexual hormones: estrogens (that characterize the female phenotype) and testosterone (which characterizes the male phenotype), which act on bone in different ways. Testosterone is the most powerful hormone in ensuring resistent and elastic bones, characteristics needed to be able to absorb shock, ie a trauma, without breaking. Resistence and elasticity are the features that oppose fractures, but testosterone also acts on muscle, promoting the development of muscle mass and the capacity for work (ie contraction) of muscle fibers. The two actions of testosterone, on bone and on muscle, accompany man throughout his life, including in old age, because there is no interruption in production, as happens with menopause. Even in cases of primitive or secondary hypogonadism, there remains at least some androgen production, and bone metabolism is retained; by contrast, in cases of castration of individuals guilty of sex crimes, the scientific literature reports a weakening of the skeleton. Estrogens have a completely different biological action: it acts on bone, but not on muscle, and is often produced on a reduced scale, owing to common conditions such as the removal of an ovary due to cysts, or in the course of a hysterectomy, or reduced production in post-menopause. This marks a crucial difference for the health of bones in women, and suggests that all possible attention should be paid to it.

Let us now turn to the natural history of calcium absorption in bones in the presence of adequate amounts of the key factors: sun, calcium from food, and estrogens.

In a woman's lifespan, her evolution reflects variations in estrogens: up to the age of 20, there is maximum uptake, which continues to a lesser degree up until age 30, when the accumulated calcium starts to be slowly lost. During the menopausal transition, the amount of calcium that is lost increases suddenly, as a result of fluctuation in the estrogens in the bloodstream; when estrogen values stabilize, calcium loss from the bones also slows down, although it continues for the rest of one's life. The metabolic reality is undeniable, and explains why elderly people are so susceptible to bone conditions which, as well as fractures from minimal traumas, also include posture-related deformities and instability, the prime cause of low back pain.

What can we do to limit the damage of an event that the extension of the human lifespan makes increasingly serious and disabling?

The first step is to safeguard what facilitates positive factors, ie exposure to the sun, albeit with the necessary precautions, together with a diet that includes milk and our wonderful cheeses, to ensure calcium intake, and adequate physical activity that makes demands on muscle and bone at the same time. With the transition of menopause, taking soya isoflavones (phytoestrogens) helps bones to fix calcium, combating, albeit blandly, its reduction in the organism. Much more effective is hormone replacement therapy, the role of which is widely acknowledged.

Today people are still unused to thinking that physical exercise may provide so many benefits to bone metabolism and – something not to be overlooked! – that it helps cognitive functions. Race walking, or brisk walking, is the real great remedy, because the constant, regular movement encourages calcium absorption. When women arrive at menopause, they ought to devote an hour a day to brisk walking, without citing the excuse that "we're always on the go", because occasional walking does not have the same benefits!

With a view to long-term prevention, one must remember that maximum calcium absorption occurs in the first 20 years of life, and thus it is advisable to begin regular physical activity right from adolescence, and keep it up throughout adulthood, in order to store up the largest possible reserves of calcium, to be made use of when it begins to run short.

Hormonal effects on cerebral function

Sleep disorders

Sleep disorders are common, affecting around 30% of the adult population (male and female). Sufferers have difficulty in falling asleep, they wake up repeatedly during the night, or early in the morning, and they do not feel rested after having slept. This condition seems to be influenced by aging, alcohol or drug abuse, major life changes, depression, low socioeconomic status, health problems and the female gender[8].

---

8 Nowakowski, Meers, Heimbach, *Sleep and women's health,* in "Sleep Med. Res.", vol. 4, 2013 pp. 1–22.

The sleep cycle includes a phase of light sleep, a phase of deep sleep, and a short period called REM (*rapid eye movement*), which come one after the other, several times during the night. The greatest rest takes place in the phases of deep sleep, while REM sleep is connected to a positive mood and better brain function. This cyclical pattern changes with aging, when the phases of light sleep become dominant, losing the ability to provide rest.

The difference between the sexes as regards sleep patterns and sleep quality is noted especially in the years of perimenopause. Sleep can be affected by a variety of disorders that derive from the socio-relational sphere, but men seem to transfer their problems to sleep a lot less than women do, including women in fertile years. Indeed, we know that young women who suffer from premenstrual syndrome have great difficulty in falling asleep, and also getting enough sleep; pregnant women also have difficulty in falling asleep, tend to wake up during the night, and remain dozy during the day; as pregnancy advances, the situation gets worse, especially if there is any anxiety or depression[9]. In menopause, sleep is influenced by changes in the hormonal balance, and also by more generic aging factors, such as changes in the circadian rhythms, one's state of health, and unsuitable daily habits. In the distressing accounts that we hear from patients talking about their sleepless nights, there is probably also a touch of anxiety, and feelings linked to uneasiness over the symptom itself. Waking up during the night, which generally happens as a result of hot flashes, is very irritating, but the changes to the architecture of sleep, and losing hours of sleep, do not seem to be major events, in many cases. Insomnia represents a problem for 40–60% of women; in 26% of women in perimenopause, owing to difficulties in their daily and working life, with an obvious decline in their sense of well-being. The consequences of sleep are serious to health and

---

9 Polo-Kantola, Aukia, Karlsson H., Karlsson L., Paavonen, *Sleep quality during pregnancy: associations with depressive and anxiety symptoms*, in «"Acta Obstet. Gynecol. Scand."», vol. 96, 2017, pp. 198–206.

mood, because they make patients more vulnerable emotionally and physically[10]. Metabolic stress makes vasomotor symptoms worse, and, in the long run, leads to hypertension, diabetes and depression. Nevertheless, it seems that women who develop insomnia in this period have been susceptible ever since their youth to everything that interferes with quality of sleep. In the general population, around 28–35% of young women have difficulties linked to sleep, and are 3.5 times more likely, compared to those who get a good night's sleep, to develop a full-scale sleep disturbance, once they reach menopause[11]. According to many women's experience, the quality of sleep gets worse during the transition to menopause, in other words in the years preceding and following the last menstruation. Alongside women in whom the characteristics of sleep go hand-in-hand with the appearance and worsening of hot flashes, there are patients for whom insomnia is the main disturbance, remaining constant over the years, while vasomotor symptoms are only mild, and transient. The typical picture of insomnia includes repeatedly waking up during the night at least three nights a week, although not all women are the same, and there is a lot of variability in the picture that we find. Those most affected not only wake up during the night, but also experience difficulty in getting to sleep, find themselves waking up too early, and experience more frequent hot flashes.

Both the quality of sleep described by patients and its architecture, which can be traced from polysomnograms[12], suggest that

---

10 Zaslavsky, LaCroix, Hale, Tindle, Shochat, *Longitudinal changes in insomnia status and incidence of physical, emotional, or mixed impairment in postmenopausal women participating in the Women's Health Initiative (WHI) study*, in "Sleep Med.", vol. 16, 2015, pp. 364–71.

11 Freeman, Sammel, Gross, Pien, *Poor sleep in relation to natural menopause: A population based 14-year follow up of midlife women*, in "Menopause", vol. 22, 2015, pp. 719–26.

12 Polysomnography is the recording of physiological parameters during the night.

the causes of insomnia display an association between the effects of aging, such as instability of the circardian rhythms, and the effects of menopause, such as hot flashes, night sweats, and frequent awakenings. In women who are overweight, or actually obese, both in their fertile years and in menopause, the characteristics of sleep obtained with home polysomnography show that the distribution of abdominal fat, or the presence of the metabolic syndrome, were associated with high fragmentation of the circadian rhythms. By comparison with women in premenopause, those in postmenopause had less stability in their circadian rhythms, and greater anomalies in their sleep architecture.[13]

It can be hard for the doctor to work out the specific cause of insomnia in a female patient, because the subjective symptoms are a reflection of both vasomotor disorders and mood disturnaces. Hot flashes go hand-in-hand with waking up at night, with sleep that is not rest-giving, daytime sleepiness, and reduced functional capabilities, leading to scenarios that can largely overlap; but one revealing difference is that depression is marked by a difficulty in falling asleep, and by the fact of waking up too early, while hot flashes lead to waking up repeatedly during the night.

Hormones and sleep disturbances

Although sleep disturbances are frequent events in women of all ages, and are part of the aging process, it is not yet clear whether, at menopause, their predominant causes are hormonal changes, vasomotor symptoms, anxiety or depressive traits, or altered breathing patterns. Estrogens and progesterone are associated with sleep disruption during reproductive life and pregnancy;

---

13 Gomez-Santos, Saura, Lucas, Castell, Madrid, Garaulet, *Menopausal status is associated with circadian- and sleep-related alterations*, in "Menopause", vol. 23, 2016, pp. 682–90.

the circadian rhythm of cortisol, known as the stress hormone, is related to awakening, as its secretion peak occurs in the early hours of the day[14]. In turn, ovarian steroid secretion is in synchrony with the circadian rhythm of sleep, while prolactin secretion is sleep-dependent. Polysomnography has shown that changes in sleep architecture occur during the phase preceding that of the menstrual cycle (known as the luteal phase), occurring hand-in-hand with a rise in body temperature. It is evident that ovarian steroids are involved in difficulties in sleeping in menopause which, in turn, correlate with hot flashes and sweating, which are a result of a decline in estrogen levels, in an interdependent circular relationship. We know that ovarian steroids are involved in the occurrence and resolution of breathing disorders, but the mechanism whereby they come into play in the overall process of insomnia is not yet known[15]. Melatonin takes part in the regulation of the sleep/wakefulness cycle, and its secretion by the pituitary is stimulated by the dimming of light intensity. With aging, the circadian rhythm of its secretion is reduced and changed, contributing to the onset of sleep disorders. The levels of melatonin decline particularly during menopause, but their influence on sleep is determined by individual characteristics. Indeed, melatonin secretion in response to the dimming of light remains essentially the same in postmenopausal women who do not have sleep problems, while its production is lower, and delayed by around fifty minutes, in a woman with a disorder. This would indicate that it is not menopause in itself that alters the melatonin cycle, but a genetic predisposition that is facilitated by the advent of menopause, but affecting only one section of the population. The circadian clock undergoes important changes during the lifespan of every individual, male or female. One

---

14 Teran-Perez, Arana-Lechuga, Esqueda-Leon *et alii*, Hormones and sleep regulation, in "Mini Rev. Med. Chem.", vol.12, 2012, pp. 1040–1048.

15 Epson, Purdie, *Effects of sex steroids on sleep*, in "Ann. Med.", vol. 31, 1999, pp. 141–145.

example is the disruption of the sleep/wakefulness rhythms that occurs as one ages, rhythms connected to the reduced endogenous production of melatonin. This phenomenon is particularly evident during menopause, and affects all women. However, not all women suffer from it in the same way, because individual sensibility to biological processes is different.

How can sleep disorders be dealt with in women in menopause?

Insomnia, as a passing, repeated event, strikes most women during menopause. For some, it is a completely new symptom, while for others it represents the worsening of a function that has always been compromised.

Insomnia can be tackled in many ways, ranging from lifestyle changes to an array of medicines; naturally, each of these remedies will be more or less suited to one woman or another; in any event, behavioral interventions are often more effective than medicines, and represent the forefront of treatment; they ought to be administered first, always. Of course, even before thinking about how to treat a patient, it is necessary to know her medical history in order to take action on possible organic conditions involved in the onset of insomnia. These include chronic pain conditions, breathing disorders, incontinence, depression, and anxiety neurosis, which require specific forms of medical intervention.

Behavioral therapy interventions specifically designed to foster sleep are regarded as the first-choice form of treatment, able to maintain good results in the long term, compared with medication, which acts immediately, but is addictive. Another advantage not to be underestimated is that these interventions can also be suggested to people who have concomitant conditions, both organic and psychiatric, although not so serious as to prevent normal daily activities. The suggested strategies include interventions in lifestyle, in the environment, and on behavior.

When it comes to lifestyle changes that can be suggested, moderate physical activity has shown itself to be effective in improving the quality of sleep in sedentary people. Work programs of 2 to 4 hours a week, comprising activities such as yoga, aerobics, active walking and generic strengthening exercises, lead to a significant improvement, that can be appreciated by the patient in terms of an increased sense of well-being[16]. Attention to mealtimes and type of diet also has a certain importance: Not having heavy meals, avoiding coffee, and not drinking too much alcohol immediately before going to bed is a commonsense rule that everyone ought to observe, but it becomes more important in people whose sleep is particularly fragile. Other suggestions relate to the need to let go of the worries of the day, not working or watching television in bed, interrupting daily activities for something that is a good preparation for sleep (like an herbal infusion or a bath), choosing a dark room, far from outside noises and not too heated, but especially establishing a habit of going to sleep at a time in keeping with the rhythms of life, and strenuously sticking to these rituals. Obviously, activities incompatible with sleep, activities that increase mental excitement or muscular work, are to be avoided in these patients, while they might be completely neutral in people who do not suffer from insomnia. Intervening in one's behavior requires a commitment to maintaining a strict time for going to bed, and an equally strict time for getting up, and not staying in bed beyond the agreed time, avoiding naps, and keeping an accurate diary for recording daily variations. Carefully compiling a diary is a commitment that the patient makes with herself to keep a watch on any "bending of the rules" in her behavior, and to record her progress. Negative thoughts, levels of attention and concerns over sleep can be noted down and discussed with the therapist.

---

16 Hartescu, Morgan, Stevinson, *Increased physical activity improves sleep and mood outcomes in inactive people with insomnia: A randomized controlled trial*, in "J. Sleep Res.", vol. 24, 2015, pp. 526–534.

Prescriptions are built around cognitive mechanisms: not staying in bed when awake serves to associate the bed only with sleeping time; relaxing activities interrupt worries over not being able to sleep and stimulate pleasant thoughts; getting out of bed (and trying again later) if one has not fallen asleep after half an hour serves to interrupt obsessive thoughts about not managing to sleep.

The external contribution of hormones such as melatonin or estrogen and progesterone, in various combinations, is used in treating insomnia. Of these, probably the most effective and most often used treatment is based on ovarian steroids, acting on the phenomenon of broken nights and hot flashes, at one and the same time. Giving exogenous ovarian hormones seems most effective for reducing sleep disorders, using formulations in low doses that can be administered in various different ways. Taking estrogen improves quality of sleep, but it is not clear whether its mechanism of action acts directly on the architecture of sleep or on reducing hot flashes and regulating the breathing pattern[17].

Despite its effectiveness, hormone replacement therapy is not suitable for all women. It has contraindications in patients with an increased risk of cancer, who have to be advised directly by their specialist about whether or not it is appropriate to take these drugs. It should be noted that the most important negative side effect that must be considered by every woman is that estrogens encourage blood coagulation and increase the risk of thrombosis, including oral contraceptives, and so patients with a personal predisposition or family history of episodes of thrombosis will have to consider other formulations.

Melatonin has a positive influence on the sleep/wakefulness cycle. It makes one feel drowsy, and reduces the time it takes to

---

17 Moline, Brooch, Zak, Gross, *Sleep in women across the life cycle from adulthood through menopause*, in "Sleep Medicine Reviews", vol. 7, 2003, pp 155–177.

fall asleep after lying down in bed in patients with insomnia. The drug reduces the number of times a patient wakes up at night, and, if need be, it can be used in association with hormonal medications. Moreover, it does not have side effects such as headaches or drowsiness, which are common in the case of many other drugs, and it seems suitable for prolonged use.

Antidepressants in low doses are used to alleviate sleep disorders in women who do not have signs of depression (which, if present, would require a different pharmacological approach). Among the more recently formulated antidepressants, low doses seem equally effective in improving the quality of sleep after three months of treatment. The medical literature presents results that are not always uniform regarding the effectiveness of antidepressants, but their use may be considered in cases where other drugs are not advisable.[18]

Sleeping pills (anxiolytics, sleep-inducing drugs, and sedatives) are drugs more suited for temporary use than ongoing use, since they may have side effects, and may cause drowsiness during the daytime, and an addiction that restricts their effectiveness. The best use of them is in treating a temporary episode of insomnia. What's more, they may have side effects, and their sedative action does not seem specific for sleep disorder in menopause.[19]

Albeit with the necessary precaution in long-term prescription, sleeping pills have been used extensively since the 1950s by a huge number of patients, offering significant improvement in the quality of sleep, in terms of both reducing the time it takes to fall asleep and reducing broken sleep, and as an increase in the

---

18 Attarian, Hachul, Guttuso, Phillips, *Treatment of chronic insomnia disorder in menopause: Evaluation of literature,* in "Menopause", vol. 22, 2015, pp. 674–684.

19 *Ibidem.*

total number of hours slept; their most frequent side effect is residual drowsiness the following morning[20].

Acupuncture seems effective in the short term for treating insomnia linked to menopause. Ten-session cycles of acupuncture, carried out in the space of three weeks, have significantly improved the effectiveness of sleep in line with the parameters of the number of hours slept, and the fact the patient wakes up less often during the night. Acupuncture also seems effective in cases of intractable insomnia, especially resistent to every approach in traditional Western medicine[21].

Over-the-counter drugs

Valerian is an extract from two plants, *Valeriana officinalis* and *Valeriana edulis*, and it is available in various formulas that may contain different concentrations of the active principle. Studies of the effectiveness of valerian on sleep have shown uncertain or conflicting results, with minimal effectiveness of the formulation compared to a placebo; its side effects are also similar to a placebo, and there is no residual drowsiness. Despite the fact there are no studies that analyse the effects of taking it over a prolonged period, the lack of adverse effects means that the drug is considered in the case of older or more fragile patients.

---

20 Schroeck, Ford, Conway *et alii, Review of safety and efficacy of sleep medicines in older adults*, in "Clinical Therapeutics", vol. 38, 2016, pp. 2340–2372.

21 Fu, Zhao, Liu *et alii, Acupuncture improves peri-menopausal insomnia: A randomized controlled trial*, in "Sleep", vol. 40, 2017. Li, Lu, *Clinical observation on acupuncture treatment of intractable insomnia*, in "Journal of Traditional Chinese Medicine", vol. 30, 2010, pp. 21–22.

Mood changes, depression and anxiety

Depression, in its various stages of severity, is a widespread disorder affecting twice as many women as men; throughout one's life, the chance of developing a major depressive disorder is 10 to 25% for women, and 5 to 12% in men. The first episode occurs around age 20, and recurrences are variable; in some cases, many months elapse from one episode to the next, in other cases two or three episodes are repeated soon after each other, and as one gets older the frequency tends to increase. Forty percent of patients who have had their first ever episode will have a recurrence within the year, and 50–60% of them should expect a further episode, with a 70% chance of having others in the years to follow. When a major depression occurs for the first time in adult life, it is often triggered by a severe psychosocial event, such as the death of a loved one, a diagnosis of a potentially fatal disease, or a divorce. Scientific studies suggest that stress has a role in precipitating the first or the second episode, but not subsequent ones. The disorder tends to run in the family, and is 1.5-3 times more frequent in the parents or children of people who are ill than in the general population, but it is not in relation with ethnic group, level of education, or socioeconomic status.

In clinical settings, the word depression is often used in a general sense, to indicate a non-specific emotional disturbance, a downcast mood, and some difficulties in daily relationships, symptoms which are very different from the more severe condition of major depressive disorder.

Depression and menopausal transition

At a time as fragile as menopausal transition, it may happen that many women display signs that suggest a state of depression: a greater tendency to get tired and irritable, and more difficulty in remaining active and maintaining concentration, along with changes in mood, appetite, and sleep patterns. Against this background, anxiety, which always accompanies depression, also increases: She becomes more worried over the things that need to be done, and family organization, and above all for loved ones. Specifically, episodes of unstable mood are relatively common, with a frequency from 2 to 14 times greater than in other moments, and with 75% of women developing hyperreactivity or hypersensibility to unfavorable psychosocial conditions.[22]

In the period of the perimenopause, psychcological distress manifests itself more frequently, and there is an increased risk of an initial episode of depression, or a recurrence of it. Why is this? The cause lies in the mutual influence of various different elements, which are all linked to mood changes. The hormonal balance of menopause, the ability to react to a difficulty, social support, lifestyle and the occurrence of a stressful event become interwoven with each other in a complex way, and the balance between them determines a person's emotional well-being. Although we rarely find ourselves dealing with full-scale, clinical depression, one must be careful in correctly evaluating a patient's distress, because differential diagnosis is not simple. Indeed, as many doctors know from firsthand experience, it can be difficult to grasp the clinical differences between a mood change that is a reaction to changes in the menopausal transition, that is set to resolve itself, and a state of anxiety or depression that is pre-existing, and intrinsic to the person, and that is accentuated by the pyschosocial stress in this period, and that risks being prolonged. Key symptoms such as an unstable mood, insomnia and difficulty in concentration are common to both conditions, which must be recognized, to make sure that an overlooked psychological condition does not become more serious. The awareness that in the last few years we have been seeing an increased incidence of the psychological condition acts as a spur for timely intervention by the doctor. Going by the statistics in

---

22 Soares, *Menopausal transition and depression: who is at risk and how to treat it?*, in "Expert Rev Neurother", vol. 7, 2007, pp. 1285–93.

the literature, it seems that 26–33% of women develop clinical symptoms of depression, and that full-blown depression strikes 12–23% of them. The association between menopause and psychopathology is a result, on the one hand, of physical stresses such as hot flashes and insomnia that alter the sleep pattern and cause discomfort, making it impossible to recoup energy; on the other hand, it is also a result of sources of psychosocial stress, such as retirement, financial hardship, and a decline in one's physical capabilities. Some studies show that depression is more frequent during the menopausal transition than at any other time, regardless of insomnia, hot flashes or anything else. This seems especially true for women who have suffered from it previously; indeed, together with a family history, previous clinical experience of depression is the most important predictive factor; by the same token, it is unlikely that the first episode of major depression will be presented at this time, unless serious traumatizing events take place. Despite the fact that clinical observations do not always agree with each other, all studies show that vulnerability is manifested in the transition period, and not when menopause is stabilized[23].

It is significant that mood changes are more frequent when there are concomitant events in reproductive life marked by specific hormonal changes, as in the pre-menstrual phase, in the *post partum* period, and at menopause. Pre-menstrual syndrome strikes 3–5% of women, and is characterized by a depressive trait, marked anxiety, an unstable mood, and a loss of interest that develops in the last part of the menstrual cycle, and which are repeated for several months in a row. The symptoms disappear at the start of menstruation, and do not present again until the days leading up to the following cycle. Postpartum depression is presented within four weeks after giving birth, with a frequency of 1 in every 500 to 1 in every 1,000 births, and preferentially affects women

---

23 Freeman, *Associations of depression with the transition to menopause*, in "Menopause", vol. 17, 2010, pp. 823–7.

who have suffered depression, or who have a family history of the illness. The symptoms include especially an unstable mood, acute anxiety, uncontrollable crying and feelings of guilt, or a lack of interest in the newborn baby.

A larger number of patients, around 20%, develop a pattern of anxiety in the absence of symptoms of full-scale depression. This can happen later on, within the first year after the baby's birth, with symptoms such as apprehension, insomnia and irritability, which go beyond the normal stress of becoming a parent. The state can be serious enough to interfere with taking care of the baby, and such as to require medical intervention.[24]

Menopausal transition is marked by endocrine fluctuations, because the balance between the hormones in the bloodstream is altered. This series of events, occurring one after the other, represents a real source of irritation for the emotional vulnerability of patients who are predisposed toward it[25]. One should note that mood changes appear more accentuated the bigger the hormonal fluctuations, also when one compares people with a differing predisposition, constituting a stress for the cognitive processes, including short-term memory. By contrast, the phases of life in which hormonal production remains stable, although reduced, as happens in stabilized menopause, seem less susceptible to mood changes.

Who is at risk?

Irritability, pronounced self-criticism, and intolerance towards menopause are traits found in women most susceptible to depression. This period is marked by a rise in irritability, even when a suitable mood is maintained; deterioration of mental equilibrium

---

24 Toler, *et Al., Screening for postpartum anxiety: A quality improvement project to promote the screening of women suffering in silence* in "Midwifery", vol. 62, 2018, pp. 161–170.

25 See note 20.

is 2–4 times more frequent than in reproductive age, even among women who had never been anxious or depressed before, precisely because hormone fluctuations represent a factor of biological vulnerability that lowers the threshold of irritability, to the point of contributing to the onset of depression[26].

Life events and previous experiences can lead to a risk of developing a deteriorated mood, albeit outside the limits of full-scale depression. Personal health problems, or relatives' health problems, a loss of interest in work, and solitude play a negative role, while the ability to overcome unpleasant events, and a satisfying lifestyle, and the fact of having maintained one's social role and network of relationships with friends and in one's family (as happens with those women who, after leaving work, find themselves even busier than before, because they take care of their grandchildren) create a sense of well-being, contribute to personal gratification, and represent a factor of protection against psychological uneasiness. If growing old successfully means adding life to one's years, and not just years to one's life, which living standards and medical progress ensure we can enjoy, then maintaining gratifying interests is the key to defeating moodiness.

How can it be treated?

If hormone fluctuations are implicated in mood instability and in the development of depression, it is plausible that taking hormones may improve one's mood more effectively than classical antidepressants.[27]

26 Mauas, Kopala-Sibley, Zuroff, *Depressive symptoms in the transition to menopause: The roles of irritability, personality vulnerability, and self-regulation*, in "Arch Womens Ment Health", vol. 17, 2014, pp. 279–289.

27 Herrera, Hodis, Mack, *Estradiol therapy after menopause mitigates effects of stress on cortisol and working memory*, in "J. Clin. Endocrinol. Metab.", vol. 102, 2017, pp. 4457–4466.

Transdermic preparations, especially, seem the best for stabilizing concentrations of hormones, combating the onset of depressive traits, and even alleviating the symptoms of major depression.

Metabolic changes

Metabolic syndrome is constituted by a set of clinical characteristics that include abdominal obesity, alterations in the lipid profile, hypertension and diabetes, conditions that are different, but interdependent. Together, these alter the state of health and make the patient more susceptible to cardiovascular disease. The appearance of the syndrome in women in reproductive age is favored by particular endocrine states, as during pregnancy, or altered, as in the case of polycystic ovary syndrome (PCOS). It arises at menopause as a response to reduced estrogens in the bloodstream.

Hyperglycemia, hypertension, abdominal obesity and an altered lipid profile constitute risk factors for metabolic syndrome, which is diagnosed when three of these characteristics are present, and occurs with a frequency greater than 50% in women over the age of 56, whose blood pressure tends to increase with age, and in relation to the number of years since her last menstruation. Its appearance also reflects the tendency toward a sedentary lifestyle, which further promotes the accumulation of abdominal fat. It is more common in women than in men, and tends to increase as one gets older. Sex hormones regulate the deposit of fat in tissue by means of the activity of transport proteins. At menopause, the decline in estrogen reduces the availability of these proteins, increases the rate at which abdominal fat is deposited, and increases the propensity toward hyperglycemia, hypertension and altered lipid profile. Abdominal obesity affects around 72% of women after the age of 60, supports metabolic syndrome, and, in the sequence of related biochemical events it is the main cause of cardiocirculatory disease, the risk of which increases by 4 times at a distance of 10 years since the onset of menopause.

Conditions that lead to the risk of the syndrome

Metabolic syndrome and obesity are interdependent, and together they can cause considerable health problems. In this connection, an alert comes from the WHO, which shows that the increase in weight in the world's population is growing at an alarming rate. Currently 35% of adults (men and women) are overweight, and 11% are frankly obese. Body weight that is above limits determined by one's constitution and age constitutes one of the most serious dangers to health, not least of which is a predisposition to metabolic syndrome. These undeniable facts direct our attention to healthier habits, not only based on a careful diet but also involving constant physical activity, the effectiveness of which is unquestioned in combating the onset of diabetes and cardio-circulatory conditions.

Unfortunately, recommendations by themselves are not effective in changing people's habits, and the remedies, however simple, are not easy to follow without professional help and support from the nearest social environment. A small group of women friends who support each other when they decide to change their eating habits, or a lady who finds empathy in her family to change her lifestyle, will have far greater chances of success than someone embarking on this change by herself.

Possible factors leading to an early appearance of the syndrome

Metabolic syndrome originates from a reduction of estrogens in the bloodstream, linked to the age at which menopause arrives; in turn, this is determined by genetic factors and aspects of lifestyle, such as diet, smoking, socioeconomic conditions, the use of oral contraceptives, and the presence of chronic metabolic illnesses. It is not clear whether the age of menopause is also connected to conditions such as eating disorders, ovarian or cardiocirculatory conditions, and hypertension. Since it depends on estrogen reduction, metabolic syndrome is also presented in young women who entered early menopause for whatever reason, and it is important to be aware of this in order to intervene in time in health problems that would be unexpected in an age bracket younger than age 50. For younger women, medical conditions are exacerbated by a psychological state made fragile by the negative experience of untimely menopause.

The medical conditions that contribute in bringing forward menopause are:

1. Taking antidepressants that alter ovarian endocrine production (although research findings do not always agree).

2. Diabetes acting differently depending on the age at which it occurs: child diabetes, diagnosed before age 20, correlates with the early onset of menopause, while later diabetes is not; it should be borne in mind that diabetes and menopause take a few years to manifest, and affect the same age group. The biochemical mechanism of the two conditions means it is not possible to establish whether, or in what sequence, one condition contributed to the development of the other.

3. Some gynecological operations completely deprive the organism of the amount of estrogens produced in menopause, and increase the risk of coronary disease and osteoporosis. Even when the ovaries are retained, the anatomy of the circulatory system is altered, owing to indirect damage due to ablations and cauterizations. The reduced blood flow is sufficient to have a negative impact on ovarian function, and to trigger early menopause.

CHAPTER 3

Menopause and Sexual Desire Disorders

How desire changes

Many women who have a happy relationship desire a sex life that is active, lively, and varied just as much as their men do, contrary to popular anecdotes. Unfortunately, we often note that, over the years, female desire evolves in a way that is not exactly positive. The waning of erotic interest has little to do with the quality of the relationship; indeed it occurs despite the gratification of sharing one's life with one's partner. To the superficial observer it may be hard to understand why this happens, but for women who are more aware the reason is clear. Performing the many roles that fall on their shoulders, being a wife, a mother, a homemaker, a worker, and a source of support for the expanded family, absorbs one's energies and suffocates eroticism. Feeling that one is a prisoner of these roles, along with the loss of romantic play, too much familiarity and the desexualization of interaction with one's husband dulls erotic sensations and extinguishes the spark that makes a woman feel seductive.

This relational and social mechanism develops independently alongside the physical changes of menopause, but comes on top of them.

Menopause occurs around age 50, and in the following decade those alterations of the organism become evident, those changes that result from endocrine changes, aging, and the side effects of common conditions for this age group. Some of these may have sexual implications, although most of the dysfunctions do not have organic causes. In particular, the loss of estrogens in the bloodstream, which is a typical symptom of menopause, changes the turgidity and tone of the genitals, mood alterations act on sexual interest, a hysterectomy[28] (very frequent around the age of 50) can change feelings about sex, while tumors, which today allow a long survival, have an impact on mood and on romantic relationships.

One positive note is that social acceptance toward sexuality among older people has increased a lot in the last 30 years, hand-in-hand with the fact that today more than 50% of women in their 70s are active, as against 30% in the past; this constitutes positive support for erotic expression, on condition, of course, that vaginal dryness, urinary incontinence, prolapse and symptoms of depression are kept under control.

Vaginal atrophy and genito-urinary syndrome

The reduction of estrogens in the bloodstream acts on the tissues of the vulva and vagina with an action which, unlike hot flashes, becomes evident only years later, and comes on top of the physiological processes of aging. With differing intensities, it affects around 80% of postmenopausal women and leads to troublesome symptoms, although there is rarely an actual set of true, painful symptoms[29]. Here we are looking at dryness, itching and dyspareunia (pain during the sexual act), which are located in the external genitals, together with a greater frequency and urgency of urinating, and a rise in infections, with their associated set of symptoms. The characteristic appearance of the external genitals shows a thinning of the pubic hair, the labia majora become less swollen, and the labia minora become thinner. An internal examination allows the gynecologist to check on other

---

28 Surgical technique to remove the uterus.
29 Kingsberg, Krychman, Graham, *et alii, The women's empower survey: Identifying women's perceptions on vulvar and vaginal atrophy and its treatment*, in "J. Sex. Med.", vol. 14, 2017, pp. 413–424.

signs caused by the aging process, such as loss of elasticity in the walls, and the thinning of the mucous lining of the vaginal canal. Following hormonal changes, there is a reduced production of lactic acid, and as a result a vaginal pH that offers less protection against bacteria and microrganisms. This makes older women more subject to vaginal and urinary infections, just like girls before their first menstrual cycle, because they are both almost wholly without estrogens.

The atrophic mucosa impacts psychophysical well-being, because, in response to the erotic stimulus, it does not lubricate the area very much and compromises sexual capability; indeed, the reduced amount of mucous is not enough to protect the delicate vaginal tissues from the rubbing action of the penis, leading to pain, with burning sensations, followed by anxiety, discomfort, and a negative expectation that can interfere with fantasy, desire, excitement and pleasure. Obviously this compromises one's sex life, and the couple's relationship. Luckily, in most cases, the pain from rubbing can be alleviated with local and general medication. For more serious forms, behavioral sexual therapy can be suggested.

The urinary tract develops from the same embryonic tissue as vaginal tissue, and for this reason it suffers in an equally negative way from estrogen reduction[30]. The loss of elasticity comes on top of the general aging process characterized by the loss of muscle tone and by birth traumas that only become evident years later. Together, they cause incontinence, with difficulty in urine retention, and involuntary urine loss, affecting around 50% of elderly women[31]. This happens because the loss of tone in the muscles and tissues is no longer able to counter the abdominal pressure which increases with sneezing, coughing, bending over to pick up heavy objects such as a laundry basket or shopping bag,

30 Sadler T., *Embriologia Medica di Langman*, Piccin Editore, 1972.
31 Khazali, Hillard, *The postmenpausal bladder*, in "Obstet., Gynaecol. and Repr. Med.", vol. 19, 2009, pp. 147–151.

or even just a sudden laugh. When risk factors are present such as advanced age, obesity, or birth traumas, which further reduce muscle tone, the ability to compensate for intra-abdominal pressure is diminished, and the clinical situation appears more serious, to the extent that one is not even able to control the normal pressure of a full bladder, and there is a continual "dripping" that is hard to control, causing a bad smell, and this is a source of understandable awkwardness in social interactions. Continual contact with acidic urine also creates micro-lesions that causes a burning sensation in the delicate tissues of the external genitals, completing a situation of considerable discomfort and functional limitation.

Estrogen receptors are found in the bladder, urethra, vaginal mucous and support structures such as the uterosacral ligaments, the levator ani and the pubococcygeus. The whole of the urinary tract is affected by the loss of estrogens, and this explains why, in 70% of cases, incontinence presents after menopause. The condition strikes women twice as often as men, and is associated with a worsening of the quality of life and of specific health conditions. Its frequency in the general population is set to rise, because it is directly linked to aging, which alone constitutes the biggest risk factor for this pathology. With aging there is a reduction in bladder capacity, the perception of the sensation of a full bladder and the resistance of the urethra, along with the innervation of the detrusor muscle. Episodes of incontinence directly affect a patient's everyday activities, because they force her to always have a toilet nearby, or else risk passing water involuntarily in public, with understandable embarrassment, and lead to broken nights, interspersed with frequently having to get up to go to the bathroom[32].

Clinical observation is backed up by studies on animals that have shown that hormone deprivation causes a gradual reduction

---

32 Natalin, Lorenzetti, Dambros, *Management of OAB in those over age 65*, in "Curr. Urol. Rep.", vol. 14, 2013, pp. 379–385.

of the muscle fibers and collagen in the support tissues, which become weaker, and therefore contribute to incontinence. However, unlike what happens with the genitals, urinary disorders do not respond well to hormone replacement therapy (see previous chapter); local treatment with estrogens improves the collagen content of the support structures, and the degree of atrophy in the structures of the lower genital tract, but it is not very effective, and is not always recommended in treating incontinence. Instead, recommended ways of treating incontinence involve behavioral changes, bladder exercises, and pelvic floor exercises, in the case of a moderate condition, and patients who are able to follow instructions. More invasive interventions, from pharmacological treatment to surgery, are reserved only for the most serious cases[33].

Mood disorders and sexuality

Interest in sex is a natural instinct that is vital for the survival of the species. In humans, this instinct responds to conditions such as a sense of well-being and romantic gratification. During one's lifespan, states such as being in love enhance it, while others, such as illness, discord, or mood disorders suppress it. Depression, in different forms and to differing degrees, frequently arises at the menopausal transition, whether it is a first episode caused by the hereditary nature of the illness, or a repetition of previous episodes as regards the severest forms. With a rise in the incidence, the fact that depression has a major impact on one's sex life becomes clear, while other causes that become more frequent at menopause are forms of physical stress, such as insomnia and

---

33 Burgio, *Update on behavioral and physical therapies for incontinence and overactive bladder*, in "Curr. Urol. Rep.", vol. 14, 2013, pp. 457–464. Hersh, Salzman, *Clinical management of urinary incontinence in women*, in "Am. Fam. Physician", vol. 87, 2013, pp. 634–640.

hot flashes, and forms of emotional stress such as bereavement, loneliness, and financial hardship in the case of less severe forms.

The word *depression* may be understood and used in many different ways: it may refer to a normal emotion, to a clinical symptom or a pathology. In the general sense, it means a worsening of optimal cognitive perception, and a mood fluctuation in daily life, but within characteristics of normality; feeling sad, discouraged, and disappointed is part and parcel of life's ups and downs.

By contrast, *Major Depressive Disorder* is an important condition that is manifested with a desire to isolate oneself, difficulty in concentrating, insomnia, and loss of appetite and of interests, in particular an interest in sex[34]. The connection between a psychiatric disorder and the loss of sexual desire is so direct that it constitutes one of the stable diagnostic criteria for depression. Indeed, we refer to "anhedonia" as the inability to experience pleasure in all or almost all activities, including sexual satisfaction. Proof of this lies in the observation that, in patients who turn to a sexual medical service, a high incidence of depression is found, which was not diagnosed prior to the appearance of a sexual dysfunction[35]. Of all psychological difficulties, anxiety is the most powerful in blocking the erotic response, and together with depression it is the most significant factor affecting the quality of one's sex life in older age, especially for those women who have developed negative emotions and difficulty in interpersonal communication and in sharing intimacy, as a response to the changes of the menopause.

Hypoactive sexual desire disorder is another matter; this is a separate condition unto itself, and it very often presents in adulthood after a period of adequate function. It may follow stressful events or interpersonal difficulties, or be associated with a low quality

---

34 Sadock B.J., Sadock V.A., Benjamin et alii, *Kaplan & Sadock's Comprehensive Textbook of Psychiatry*, Williams & Wilkins, Baltimora, 1981.

35 Watson J.P., *Sexual behavior, relationship and mood*, in "British Journal of Clinical Practice", vol. 4, 1979, pp. 23–26.

of life, but in most cases there is no one cause that may justify its outbreak, nor a direct link with the menopause, or with medical or psychiatric conditions. HSDD remains relatively constant in the various age groups, being present in 8.9% of women aged between 18 and 44, in 12.3% of those aged 45–64, and in 7.4% of those older than 65[36]. The prevalence of a diminution of sexual desire, caused by many situations of discomfort and uneasiness, is as high as 43% of the general population, while the more complex disorder HSDD affects 10%[37]. It comes with an inability to have fantasies, and a loss of desire for sex, or interest in sex. This condition changes the equilibrium of a person's sex life without an apparent reason, and may be a source of distress that is profound enough to bring about the end of the relationship.

These aforementioned situations have features that are partly overlapping, but the differences are crucial: in one instance, the diminution of desire is a corollary of generalized discomfort, while in the other it is part of the diagnosis of clinical depression, and as such it is not diagnosed by itself, while HSDD is recognized as a separate clinical entity.

Hysterectomy

Simple hysterectomy is the most frequent gynecological surgical operation after a Caesarean section. It is performed on patients in various different age groups, but especially in the 10 years from age 50 to age 60, for non-cancerous conditions such as endometriosis, fibromatosis and prolapse, and it affects a considerable number of

---

36 Parish, Hahn, *Hypoactive sexual desire disorder: A review of epidemiology, biopsychology, diagnosis, and treatment*, in "Sex. Med. Rev.", vol. 4, pp. 103–120.

37 Kingsberg, Rezaee, *Hypoactive sexual desire in women*, in "Menopause", vol. 20, 2013, pp. 1284–1300.

otherwise healthy, active women. The clinical symptoms affecting all the conditions mentioned include frequent bleeding, abdominal spasms, urinary incontinence, low back pain, and dyspareunia, and in most cases they are completely resolved by the operation. Since the 1980s there has been a continual decline in its frequency, thanks to improvements in the pharmacological armamentarium, and in surgical techniques offering less invasive alternatives. Up until around 15 years ago, hysterectomies were carried out with conventional surgical techniques, and it is calculated that around one third of all women in the West over age 65 have had this operation[38]. Since the end of the 1990s the laparoscopic approach[39] has become the preferred operation, because it causes less trauma to the abdominal wall and to the pelvic organs, it stimulates fewer painful symptoms in the post-op phase, it allows prompt functional recovery and, in general, leads to fewer complications. Currently it represents the prferred method in at least 2/3 of all operations[40].

When carried out with the right indications, a hysterectomy brings an undoubted improvement in quality if life and in sexuality, because it eliminates painful symptoms. The damage once caused by techniques that were still in their infancy, such as the reduction and shortening of the vaginal canal, and the scars that once made penetration painful, if not impossible, are now things of the distant past, and must not longer be a source of concern for a woman preparing for this operation.

---

38 Wilcox, Koonin, Pokras *et alii, Hysterectomy in the United States 1988–1990,* in "Obstet. Gynecol.", vol. 83, 1994, pp. 549–555.

39 Laparoscopy is a surgical practice which avoids invasive incisions: instead, operations are performed using probes, pincers, surgical staples, etc, by means of small holes made in the abdominal wall.

40 Kreuninger, Cohen, Meurs *et Alii, Trends in readmission rate by route of hysterectomy,* in "Acta Obstet Gynecol Scand", vol. 97, 2018, pp. 285–293. Sandberg, la Chapelle, van den Tweel *et Alii, Laparoendoscopic single-site surgery versus conventional laparoscopy for hysterectomy,* in "Arc Gynecol Obstet", vol. 295, 2017 pp. 1089–1103.

A recent review of the medical literature has evaluated the effectiveness of hysterectomy as regards returning to normal activities, satisfaction, quality of life, safety against intraoperative visceral traumas and fistulas and, finally, as regards post-operative damage such as urinary and intestinal alterations, and alterations to the pelvic floor, and sexual difficulties. For this reason, gynecologists are in favour of intervention that resolves several health problems in a fairly simple way. Most patients also welcome the disappearance of gynecological symptoms in such a way as to improve well-being and, indirectly, sex. By regaining their health, patients regain their desire, and the ability to respond to erotic stimuli.

Unfortunately, this is not true in the case of all women. Some patients are unable to forget the operation they have undergone; they see it as something that has damaged their femininity, and they develop a general feeling of being upset that has repercussions on their sexual relations. The difficulty originates from non-acceptance of the surgical operation, and their image of their own body without a uterus; this leads patients to report the sensation of feeling themselves to be empty and stripped of their femininity. Thus, while most women flourish, a small number develop depression, anxiety and a loss of interest in sex. Psychotherapists, who see some patients who develop a problem, attribute many relationship and sexual problems to hysterectomies, insofar as the adverse emotional reaction to the loss of the uterus changes the body image they had of themselves and takes away their femininity, despite the undeniable improvement in their actual physical health. Since the number of hysterectomies for benign causes, and using one of a range of techniques, is huge, around 600,000 a year in the United States alone, it is vital that people in the medical profession understand the impact on the quality of life, including sexuality, of the person who undergoes this operation.

The secondary psychological effects of a hysterectomy have been studied and recognized over the course of many years. The term "post-hysterectomy syndrome" was coined more than 40 years ago, observing that women who have had a hysterectomy display greater signs of psychophysical stress and general distress than other patients who have had surgery. There is a widespread belief that both depression and sexual difficulties are based on social and cultural expectations, or that they derive from difficulties in their relationship that preceded the gynecological operation. One further possibility is that the patient already had a latent psychological difficulty or depression that only became fully manifest after the hysterectomy. Some findings tell us that a woman's attitude towards sexuality, and the gratification that is obtained from it, depend on the harmony in the relationship[41].

A particular situation which we have found in our clinical experience is represented by those women who have not fulfilled their desire to become a mother, and for whom the loss of the uterus is a signal of the impossibility of this ever happening. Patients in these studies are by definition women in menopause who are aware they have gone past the age of reproduction, but in terms of their emotional reaction only the removal of the uterus has signified to them the definitive loss of a dream.

This issue remains controversial, because one may indeed think that a hysterectomy changes the quality of the sexual relationship partly owing to psychological factors, and partly owing to the alteration of innervation and blood flow to the pelvic organs.

A reaction of psychological difficulty has been observed in a particularly high number of Asian hysterectomy patients (greater than 18%), but the significance of this statistic is hard to judge, because the psychiatric make-up of the study sample was not assessed prior to the operation itself[42]. Recent studies show that sexuality remains unchanged in a study comparing three different

41 Helström, Sörbom, Bäckström, *Influence of partner relationship on sexuality after subtotal hysterectomy*, in "Acta Obstet Scand" vol. 74, 1995, pp. 142–146.
42 Lee, Kim, Park, *Psychiatric outcome after hysterectomy in women with uterine myoma: a population-based retrospective cohort study*, in "Arch Womens Ment Health", vol. 20, 2017, pp. 487–494.

laparoscopic techniques[43], or even improves, thanks to the disappearance of symptoms, although there are a few rare cases of patients who develop an adverse reaction. In general, it seems that the quality of a sexual relationship before an operation, in terms of desire, frequency and satisfaction, may be a good predictor of what happens afterward[44].

An awareness of this potential side effect suggests it may be helpful to educate patients regarding the secondary effects of hysterectomy, so as to increase their acceptance and, ultimately, their sexual satisfaction.

Cancer conditions

The most frequent oncological conditions affect the breast, lungs, the colo-rectal tract, the uterus, the ovaries and the prostate. The incidence of tumors is especially dependent on age, and indeed we are looking at something in the region of a few dozen cases for every 100,000 individuals up to age 30, and hundreds of cases per 100,000 individuals over age 50. In the last 10–15 years a trend has been noted toward a rise in breast cancer and lung cancer for women in this age group, while tumors of the uterus and the ovaries have remained stable. The rise in occurrence that we see today is partly connected to the spread of early diagnosis, as in the case of breast conditions, and partly to a downward trend when it comes to smoking, in the case of men and women. Improvements in the process of diagnosis and treatment have proved to be effective in ensuring prolonged survival. For that

---

43 Lee, Choi, Hong et Alii, Does conventional or single port laparoscopically assisted vaginal hysterectomy affect female sexual function?, in "Acta Obstet Gynecol Scand", vol. 90, 2011, pp. 1410–1415.

44 Thakar, *Is the uterus a sexual organ? Sexual function following hysterectomy*, in "Sex Med Rev", vol. 3, 2015, pp. 264–278.

matter, the aging of the population and the reduction in mortality from other causes will increasingly lead to a higher percentage of deaths from neoplasia. As regards breast cancer, the survival rate is constantly rising, around 90% after 5 years in cases diagnosed in the last 15 years. This is thanks to early diagnosis, which is now very widespread in Italy. This detects the disease in its early stages, when it is easier to treat, and thanks to the uniform application of treatment protocols, interventions proven to be effective are possible even in outlying health centers[45].

The impact of cancer in the emotional sphere

Being given a diagnosis of neoplasia (tumor) and embarking on the necessary treatments can be devastating for a person's emotional balance, and this is often accompanied by a reaction of depression which is not restricted to the patient, but also involves her partner, too. The mood of suffering, and the physical consequences of treatment, block the couple's free expression of affection, making physical intimacy difficult and causing a suspension of sexual activity.

Usually, the first step in treating a tumor consists in surgery to remove the affected part. This is seen as a form of mutilation, with an alteration of the patient's physical appearance which, even when it is not very evident, changes her body image. When a breast is operated on, involving the symbol of feminine identity, the body image that is marred by the scar reawakens a woman's sense of shame, meaning that it becomes extremely difficult to talk about the wound. The breast is beauty, ornament and seduction, it is a source of erotic sensations and a universal symbol of motherhood; it is an integral part of the intimate image that

---

45 Istituto Toscano Tumori, *Raccomandazioni cliniche per i principali tumori solidi*, 2005.

a woman has of herself, because it is a leading player in the fundamental experiences of life.

The scars left by surgery may not be apparent in aesthetic terms, but they remain as a perpetual sign of what has happened, and may be powerful enough to prevent a woman from forgetting, even when, years later, she is clinically healed. For this reason, many women feel uncomfortable about getting undressed in front of their partner, and they don't wish their breast to be caressed. When an interest in sex does return, many of these women choose to wear underwear that conceals the affected breast, helping them to overcome their discomfort.

Longer-term emotional reactions

If patients are observed after diagnosis and initial treatment, several successive changes are seen in their emotional equilibrium in the long term, following a trajectory in which the initial anxiety turns into depression, the need to receive support increases over time, and thoughts of the illness become ever more present. Younger age and a higher degree of illness are predictors of more serious emotional distress, and a reduced ability to adapt, both personally and within the relationship.

These patients believe they get fewer benefits from treatment, and report intrusive thoughts regarding the illness, which are critical for personal motivation. Much of the impact that the tumor has on sexuality depends on the consequences of treatments that alter the hormonal, vascular and neurological systems, damaging the function and/or the anatomy of the genital organs. However, the biggest source of suffering for the patient herself, and for the couple, is the loss of well-being and independence, together with a perception of a limit set on the time she has to live. An illness that limits life, and the vision of the future, changes the response to emotional stimuli, and places a very big burden on a couple's intimacy. Indeed, we see a substantial increase in sexual dysfunctions in women who undergo a gynecological operation, or other treatments for neoplasms. Unfortunately, unless a consultancy is offered in a short space of time, it is likely that a patient will remain blocked in a pattern of avoiding sex, or dysfunctional and unsatisfactory sexuality. One year on after a breast operation, 33% of patients had suspended their sex life, having an altered body image, and a relationship in distress[46]. The patient and her partner both suffer in the same way, because they feel that their life together is placed in danger. The deep pain makes one retreat within oneself, becoming immobilized and mute, and this affects all aspects of the relationship: sharing in everyday life, displays of affection, and sexuality. To combat these limitations, a couple needs to develop a deeper intimacy, making it possible to communicate suffering in a significant way. Intimacy brings the partners closer together, combats the tendency toward isolation, and facilitates physical contact, which is the way to recoup sexuality.

Women who survive a tumor continue to suffer, because depression, physical problems and sexual difficulties continue to be present. In view of the fact that progress in medicine ensures a life expectancy, and a quality of life, that have hugely improved in just a few years, it is important that psychological support is given in the early stages of the onset of the illness, and initial treatment. It seems equally important that the partner is involved right from the start, because the couple deals with a tumor, and all that it involves, together: emotional suffering, physical problems, the change in social role, and often a renegotiation of the roles within the relationship. This last aspect is extremely delicate, because it can subvert the equilibrium of the couple and confront a person with the fact that his/her partner is no longer the person she once was. A person who used to be strong-willed and engaging may become weak and needy, while a dependent person may have

---

46 Maguire, Lee, Bevington, Küchemann et Alii, *Psychiatric problems in the first year after mastectomy*, vol. 1, 1978, pp. 963–965.

to take action, and become the strong support for everyone. The way a healthy partner supports emotional suffering constitutes a vital part of the equilibrium of the relationship, and for this reason must never be left to one side in psychological support plans[47].

The most delicate danger to the reconstruction of the intimate equilibrium of a couple is when the active treatment of the neoplasia ends, ie when the treatment protocol is completed, and there are no signs of a relapse. In this moment, there is a certain newfound freedom from medical treatment, and attention shifts to healing, although check-ups continue over the years. It is at this point that the couple reassigns new roles and new habits that developed during the years of active treatment; now intimate communication can resume, with a new confidence in the future, there is less anxiety over the illness, and sexuality finds its place again. The emotional balance improves greatly in the space of five years, but a person who had suffered in the past from depression has a higher risk of a psychological follow-on[48]. In a context of emotional suffering supported over many years, it is understandable that many women affected by breast cancer should be reluctant to talk about sex, even when it is the doctor who takes the first step. Some avoid the subject altogether, and others deny there are difficulties. These responses come from people who have faced the idea of dying, and have agreed to disabling treatments in the hope of recovery, at a time when the priority was survival, not sexuality. Luckily, intimacy and sexuality become important again as time goes by, and as physical well-being is re-established; in harmonious relationships, suffering increases intimacy and closeness to the other person, with a good erotic aspect, but a woman who has held back her romantic instinct

---

47 Di Lascio, Pagani, *Is it time to address survivorship in advanced breast cancer? A review article*. In "Breast", vol. 31, 2017, pp. 167–172.

48 Keesing, Rosenwax, McNamara, *Dyadic approach to understanding the impact of breast cancer on relationships between partners during early survivorship*, in "BMC Women's Health", 2016.

for so long, and for such serious reasons, may not be able to abandon herself to desire; the same thing happens to the partner with whom she has shared in her suffering, day after day.

Further sources of emotional stress are anger over falling ill, "Why me?", and the sadness of people who are alone, who know that they have an extra obstacle in constructing a romantic relationship. It is from these clinical observations that my own personal belief derives that sexual rehabilitation must be offered to cancer patients at an early stage, and that a door can and must be kept open to deal with dysfunctions.

Further reading:

Faubion, Sood, Kapoor, *Genitourinary syndrome of menopause*, in "Mayo Clin Proc.", vol. 92, 2017, pp. 1842–1849.

Sturdee, Panay, International Menopause Society Writing Group, *Recommendations for the management of postmenopausal vaginal atrophy*, in "Climacteric" vol. 13, 2010, pp. 509–522.

Leiblum S.R., Rosen R.C., *Principles and practice of sex therapy*, The Guilford Press, New York, 1989.

Hall K., *Reclaiming your sexual self: how you can bring desire back into your life*, John Wiley & Sons, Hoboken, 2004.

Sloan D., *The emotional and psychosexual aspects of hysterectomy*, in "Am. J. Obstet. Gynecol." vol. 131, 1978, pp. 598–605.

Linden, MacKenzie, Rnic et alii, *Emotional adjustment over 1 year post-diagnosis in patients with cancer: Understanding and predicting adjustment trajectories*, in "Support Care Cancer", vol. 23, 2015; pp. 1391–1399.

Sullivan-Singh, Stanton, Low, *Living with limited time: Socioemotional selectivity theory in the context of health adversity*, in "J. Pers. Soc. Psychol.", vol. 108, 2015, pp. 900–916.

Schover L.R., Jensen S.B., *Sexuality and the Chronic Illness*, The Guilford Press, New York, 1988.

Albaugh J., *Reclaiming Sex and Intimacy After Prostate Cancer*, Anthony J. Jannetti, Pitman, 2012.

CHAPTER 4

Romantic Relationships Among the Elderly

Psychophysical well-being

Health, in the sense of the absence of illness, is a valuable asset, but it is not sufficient to determine *well-being*, a far broader concept that includes feeling well both physically and mentally. The World Health Organization (WHO) first recognised this correspondence between the body and the psyche many years ago, and indeed in 1948 it defined well-being as "A state of complete physical, mental and social wellness, not just the absence of a state of sickness or infirmity".

In line with the spirit behind this statement, health is a positive state that enhances one's physical capabilities and personal resources. A way to think that was highly innovative for the time.

A woman's psychophysical well-being in the transition toward menopause depends on three factors: her health, her psychological equilibrium, and her level of emotional and sentimental gratification.

The former of these, health, is based on metabolic changes typical of the period. Of these, bone metabolism, vasomotor symptoms, and genital atrophy are the most evident and the ones studied most. We know that these reorganizations of organic functions are physiological, and cannot be regarded as an illness; however, they are responsible for long-term effects that present themselves as a threat to health. Fortunately, in many cases it is possible to combat the damage by carrying out preventive measures and following some "well-informed" advice to adapt one's lifestyle to the new needs.

The American College of Sports Medicine and the American Heart Association recommend that elderly people carry out moderate physical activity for 30 minutes five days a week, or vigorous activity for 20 minutes three days a week to reduce the risk of cardiocirculatory illnesses, diabetes, cancer, and osteoporosis, and to preserve mental health[49]. Obviously, in order to stay in good health, an older person must be more careful than in their youth. Unfortunately, and despite all the recommendations, women are notable by their absence in all studies on physical activity by the elderly[50]. The North American Menopausal Society offers especially specific suggestions for menopausal women, stressing that regular physical activity offers important benefits for cardiorespiratory functionality, vasomotor symptoms, cognitive function, physical equilibrium, and reducing anxiety and depression[51]. Despite the fact that most women admit that they understand the importance of staying active, and know that in so doing they would gain the approval of their family and their doctor, few of them live up to their good intentions, complaining that they have little time and too many things to do to make this commitment[52]. People who understand the impact of aging on well-being appreciate the effectivess of an innovative personal approach to prevention, and learn how to take care of themselves. The awareness of a careful lifestyle is crucial for staying in good health, makes one able to make the best decisions for

49 Nelson, Rejeski, Blair, *et al.*, *Physical activity and public health in older adults: recommendation from the American College of Sports Medicine and the American Heart Association,* in "Med Sci Sports Exerc.", vol. 116, 2007, pp. 1094–1105.

50 Booth, Owen, Bauman, *et al.*, *Social-cognitive and perceived environment influences associated with physical activity in older Australians,* in "Prev Med.", vol. 31, 2000, pp. 15–22.

51 North American Menopause Society, *Treatment of menopause-associated vasomotor symptoms: position statement,* in "Menopause", vol. 11, 2004, pp. 11–33.

52 Vallace, Murray, Johnson, *et al.*, *Understanding physical activity intentions and behaviors in postmenopausal women: an application of the theory of planned behavior,* in "Int. J. Behav. Med.", vol. 18, 2011, pp. 139–149.

oneself, and creates the motivation for transferring this knowledge to other women[53].

Psychological equilibrium evolves in response to the events of life, and to the various different phases of life.

With menopause, and with the passing of the years, everyone has to learn to live with the decline in physical and mental capacities. Women often talk about how much hot flashes, the tendency to get tired, and the difficulty in concentration interfere with their work and social life, and about the effort needed to find pleasure and curiosity in what life still offers[54].

Maintaining psychological equilibrium, in other words serenity, in the context of the sexual relationship means understanding the limitations that age brings and avoiding falling foul of unrealistic expectations, which could only lead to disappointments. There is no right way, or right frequency, for having sex, but with an open discussion every couple can establish their own style of sex, enhancing what is befitting, and what gives satisfaction. As we get older, the need for warmth and love remains high, and keeping the sexual relationship alive is a sign of adapting positively to age.

Once one's working life is over, a lot of a person's emotional and sentimental gratification depends on their family situation. The family provides a role, gives stability, and is a source of affection. The satisfaction of seeing one's role recognised by one's companion is one of the cornerstones of female psychological equilibrium. Another is represented by independence and social skills, which reinforce motivation, making it possible for a woman to perform differing roles such as mother, grandmother,

---

53 Doubova, Infante-Castañeda, Martinez-Vega, *et al.*, *Toward healthy aging through empowering self-care during the climacteric stage*, in "Climacteric", vol. 15, 2012, pp. 563–72.

54 Wodds, Mitchell, *Symptoms interference with work and relationship during the menopausal transition and early postmenopause*, in "Menopause", vol. 18, 2011, pp. 654–61.

worker, friend, and so on. By contrast, people who do not have these gratifications are more vulnerable to the difficulties, and more easily develop a decline in their psychical equilibrium[55]. Indeed, it seems very much that the sense of solitude, or satisfaction, that derives from intimate relations with one's partner and family influences well-being much more than biological factors[56].

Going back to the points made at the start of this chapter, the concept of sexual health also goes beyond the concept of the lack of a dysfunction, and in this case, too, we can draw on a WHO statement made in 1975, which described sexual health as "an integral part of general health". In 1994 the United Nations conference on population and development endorsed the right to sexual health, "the aim of which is an improvement in life, and personal relationships, and not just advice and treatment relating to reproduction and sexually-transmitted diseases"[57].

To show the holistic nature of sexual well-being, mature women who report a good level of romantic gratification are also those most motivated to engage in physical activity, who have greater social support, and who enjoy good health, and do not suffer from insomnia. Physical and emotional stimuli, which depend on lifestyle and the harmony of the couple, and the benefits of intimacy influence each other in a positive way, especially in old age[58].

Mature women engaged in the sphere of social relations maintain good emotional balance and are more satisfied by their sex

---

55 Talley, Kocum, Schlegel, et al., Social roles, basic need satisfaction, and psychological health: The central role of competence, in "Pers Soc Psychol Bull", vol. 38, 2012, pp. 155–173.

56 Fernandez-Alonso, Trabalón-Pastor, Vara, et al., Life satisfaction, loneliness and related factors during female midlife, in "Maturitas", vol. 72, 2012, pp. 88–92.

57 Cohen, Richards, The Cairo Consensus: Population, development and women, in "Fam Plan Pers", vol. 26, 1994, pp. 272–77.

58 Hess, Conroy, Ness, et al., Association of lifestyle and relationship factors with sexual functioning of women during midlife, in "J Sex Med", vol. 6, 2009, pp. 1358–1368.

life, independently of demographical factors, and whether they take hormone treatment. It is worth noting that, in women of all ages, having a purpose in life produces good psychological equilibrium, associated with happiness, satisfaction, self-esteem, self-acceptance, personal growth, and a sense of well-being and optimism[59]. Sexuality is a vital aspect of life, requiring a continual ability to change and to adapt. In order for these aspects to continue over the years, it is essential that a couple maintains physical contact in the form of caresses and hugs, and the intimacy of sincere and profound verbal communication[60]. Age increases the occurrence of difficulties in the sexual sphere, owing to the physiological processes of getting older, but low self-esteem, and less favorable circumstances, can mortify a couple more than metabolic changes, regardless of their state of health. Indeed, a minor problem may become insuperable only when a couple finds themselves living in a hostile relationship, or when there is a lack of empathy between the partners[61].

Psychological intimacy

Psychological intimacy is created when a person knows that they can talk about themselves to the other, with the certainty of finding understanding and respect. It is through emotional closeness

59 Prairie, Scheier, Matthews, Chang, *et al.*, *A higher sense of purpose in life is associated with sexual enjoyment in midlife women*, in "Menopause", vol. 18, 2011, pp. 839–844.

60 Woloski-Wruble, Oliel, Leefsma, et al., *Sexual activities, sexual and life satisfaction, and successful aging in women*, in "J Sex Med", vol. 7, 2010, pp. 2401–2410.

61 Hartmann, Philippsohn, Heiser, et al., *Low sexual desire in midlife and older women: personality factors, psychosocial development, present sexuality*, in "Menopause", vol. 11, 2004, pp. 726–740.

that gratification comes about, and sexual desire is triggered. In turn, a lively sexuality increases the motivation in discussing aspects of a relationship that may be a source of conflict such as building ties of respect, intimacy, and trust. Indeed, the successful strategy for building and maintaining a vital connection is being able to deal with differences and conflicts.

The experts say that 10–20% of conflicts cannot be resolved, in the sense that the two partners have and will continue to have differing opinions, without the possibility of a compromise that satisfies both sufficiently. Learning to accept inevitable differences, while remaining positive toward the value of one's partner, is the vital element in a circular process in which a functional relationship stimulates the best qualities and contributes to intimate emotional enrichment and sexual satisfaction.

Romantic equilibrium

The years in which a woman learns to adapt to menopause are the same that see other changes in her life, too. For most women, it is the time when they leave the world of work, and the time when grandchildren are born. The long period of menopausal transition allows a targeted adaptation of one's lifestyle, and it may be an excellent opportunity for one or two changes to the couple's contract, for the partners to reappropriate a personal space that had been sacrificed for the shared life plans. When the circumstances of work and family change, the relationship is also renewed, and the old roles evolve toward an equilibrium that reflects the experience of a shared life, while the purposes and motivations are renegotiated to reflect the evolution of the couple. Of the customary roles, the more rigid ones derive from stereotypes linked to gender, and are very hard to change, owing to the conditioning that comes from one's family and from society at large.

To imagine how the relationship of a couple on the threshold of old age may develop, let's take a long-term view. The couple, as a unit, is different from, and more complex than, the sum of the two individual people, and often reacts to a solicitation by means of mediation that incorporates the two personalities together, and indeed this privileged interaction may reveal unsuspected capabilities, characteristics and aspirations.

In the first few years, the two partners make individual decisions about what they want out of the relationship. When the relationship becomes more consolidated, from these individual positions there derives a shared intent, as when a couple, after spending time and money on themselves, wishes to start a family, and devotes their resources to looking after their children. As time goes by, the needs of the family and work responsibilities diminish, and the couple can think of themselves once again. The interaction that the couple engages in to achieve goals that are now different is the strength that changes the structure of the relationship. Indeed, when the insistent pace typical of a young family slows down, a more flexible interaction takes shape, with more nuances, allowing roles to be shared and exchanged. In the years when work commitments are to the fore, there is a tendency to divide tasks in a fairly rigid way: who deals with this, and who takes care of that, often in line with traditional roles that seem most befitting. This happens because the fact there is little time available requires optimum organization of resources and does not allow experimentation. This becomes possible, however, in the years when one is older and "freer". Dealing with housekeeping, or the family finances, for example, may involve both partners, even though up until now only one of the two has been responsible for them.

The sharing of responsibilities changes the relationship, making it less *symmetrical* and more *complementary,* and makes it easier to collaborate, or make up for the difficulties of the other; this allows greater sharing, reinforces positive emotions, satisfaction, and intimate interaction. A profound sense of reciprocity is a characteristic feature of harmonious couples. At this time of opening up and restructuring, expectations may appear on the part of one partner, for whom a compromise is necessary, because they are neither convergent nor complementary with the wishes of the other.

The fact that there may be conflicts in the transition phases should not be seen as frightening!

Quarrels and arguments represent two ways of thinking, and comparing these two ways is useful in finding a path for mediation. An argument has a great potential for positivity, because it opens the door to lively discussion and to acceptance of a different way of feeling. Clearly, acceptance of a different opinion does not mean sharing that thought; instead, it paves the way for drawing up agreed-upon solutions that would not have been possible without discussion. Differences of opinion can be accepted, even when they cannot be resolved, unless they contain elements that have a destructive effect on the relationship, whereas the real damage is done when one puts up with something in silence, just to avoid a conflict. Accepting divergences is a gift that comes from the emotional maturity of adulthood, but above all from a relationship that has kept its basic values over the years.

Relationships

After age 50, everyone has to face a worsening of one's physical condition and aesthetic appearance, the loss of one's social role that follows retirement, and the change in the structure of the family. In the third phase of life it is necessary to review the habits and values that characterized the relationship in the past, to keep what still works, and try out new paths that best suit the new pace of life and the new commitments.

In this process of restructuring, it is inevitable that the couple should face a world that has changed and the new generations who have customs and values that are hard to share in. Many couples are not free to think only of themselves, but suffer from the problematic situations of their children, now grown up but in need of their support. Despite the difficulties, usually the initial period after retirement is devoted to traveling and amusements, as if it were a second honeymoon. After a while the honeymoon ends, by definition, but a restructuring of a life of intimacy may prove to be a very engaging process. New possibilities take shape when one manages to abandon habits that are now just "empty shells" and to replace them with activities and interests that help the couple to remain connected inside a significant social support, one that offers opportunities for enrichment in the years to come.

The expectations that a person has regarding getting older are influenced by the way that they saw family members grow old, and the attitude that these family members transmitted. Metaphors and stories from one's grandparents are part of the philosophical approach to one's own aging, while from one generation to the next there remains an unchanged need to connect the present time with past time, and the need to accept the way time evolves, one of the fundamental compromises of existence[62]. It is important for the couple to understand how external pressures interfere in the relationship, and how to integrate them positively. In this period, one takes stock of previous years, and one looks ahead; when the verdict is positive, the future appears promising, but when it is not satisfying, then one's expectations also become less rosy.

Personal satisfaction is based on the two basic elements, intimate life and social life, in which there are several different components: the couple's relationship, sexuality, and one's family on one side, and work, health, success and money on the other, with the order of priorities changing depending on different people, but also in differing circumstances.

The data in the literature say that for women emotional satisfaction is influenced by psychosocial and professional aspects, and that this is reflected in the quality of communication between the partners, and equally the appreciation of one's

---

62 Papp P., *Couples on the Fault Line: New Directions for Therapists*, The Guilford Press, New York, 2000.

companion represents a major pillar for one's self-esteem. Other factors such as one's mood, the harmony of the relationship, and stressful events determine the degree of satisfaction in a direct way, independently of the hormonal variations of menopause, or the impact of hormone replacement therapy on one's sense of well-being.

In advanced age, too, the perception of well-being includes psychological, physical and sexual elements that are not restricted to the relationship, but include a sexual contact that stimulates the desire to remain connected. In women over age 65, however, the most important predictive factor of personal satisfaction depends on health and physical and mental independence, and worsens with solitude and financial problems.

As they gradually advance in years, a higher percentage of women without a stable partner live in sexual abstinence, or with few encounters per year. Between age 50 and 59, 4 out of 10 women do not have a sex life, while, after age 70, 70% do not have one, and after age 80 the percentage rises to 90%, while 60% of men of the same age, also without a stable relationship, remain active. These statistics probably do not reflect a lack of interest on the part of women, but do reflect the different value that they place on sexuality, which is seen as a source of affection and continuity in the context of an interpersonal relationship[63].

Not much is known about the sex life of elderly women, because there are not many studies of it, but it seems that today, too, the conviction that sex is unpleasant for the elderly is responsible for its decline, especially among less-educated women, who are the ones most easily influenced by the opinions of others. The fact is that it seems wrong to suppose that elderly people do not have any interest in sex; in any six-month period, more than 80% of men and women over the age of 65 have at least one romantic episode that includes expressions of sexuality and tenderness,

---

63 Michael R.T., Gagnon J.H., Laumann E.O. and Kolata G., *Sex in America*, Little, Brown and Company, London, 1994.

such as stroking and kissing. Of these, only 1–5% of women and 17% of men do not have a fixed partner[64].

Sexuality goes hand-in-hand with social support, good health, fewer symptoms of depression and a positive psychological attitude. The fact is that sexual intimacy has a role to play in the lives of many elderly couples, who remain united in the face of difficulties. The personality structure of the partners helps to determine the type of expression of sexuality and affection; indeed, couples in their 70s who present themselves in a positive way in social interactions give more importance to sex, and engage in sex more frequently than people of the same age. An attitude that is favorably disposed toward sexuality improves the quality of the relationship, and this is especially true when the male has the more extroverted character[65]. By contrast, abstinence worsens self-esteem, and undermines non-erotic moments of intimacy. As one might expect, the habits of the second half of one's life reflect those of one's previous years, but they are also the fruit of the teachings one has received. That is why older ladies, who presumably had a stricter upbringing, are more reluctant to accept a variety of sexual activities.

Sexual difficulties are present in every phase of life, and indeed 15–20% of women of all ages report one or more dysfunctions; at middle age, problems become more frequent, owing to alterations in the genital tissues, which feel the effects of the changed hormonal climate, metabolic problems, and reduced vascularization, the main damage caused by which is pain during intercourse, and difficulty in achieving orgasm. When they get old, couples who have found ways to adapt to the changes and have maintained an active sex life year after year need more than ever

64 Freak-Poli, Kirkman, De Castro Lima, *et al., Sexual activity and physical tenderness in older adults: Cross-sectional prevalence and associated characteristics*, in "Sex Med", vol. 14, 2017, pp. 918–927.

65 Waite, Iveniuk, Laumann, *et al., Sexuality in older couples: individual and dyadic characteristics*, in "Arch Sex Behav", vol. 46, 2017, pp. 605–618.

ro take advantage of their complicity to adapt their behavior to the needs of their age.

The ability to react to a condition depends on the nature of the illness, but it is also very much influenced by one's personality, by previous experiences, and by the relationship. As the years go by, the conditions and inconveniences that inevitably manifest themselves undermine serenity; maintaining an active sex life, even if it is imperfect, makes the difference in the way in which the partners succeed in managing their relationship.

Sexual health

The female sexual response feels the effects of the metabolic processes of menopause and getting old, but none of these things, by itself, constitutes an insurmountable obstacle to sexual satisfaction; however, when several elements come together, the negative effects of each are magnified, and a dysfunction is generated.

Lubrication, which allows penetration without irritation or friction, is the first thing that suffers from the hormonal climate of menopause. It is generated by the increase in blood to the genitals which, in turn, follows erotic excitement. We are looking at a mental state that changes the physical response of a part of the body. The biological phenomenon corresponds to the male erection, because it too depends on an increase in blood in the relevant organs, which is stimulated by erotic excitement. Specifically, the increased blood flow occurs in the blood vessels that supply the walls of the vagina, which are thereby elongated and lubricated to make room for the erect penis; the same vascular phenomenon in men causes the corpora cavernosa and the corpus spongiosum to fill, producing an erection that allows penetration.

The reduced blood flow owing to the mechanisms of aging makes erections less complete, and vaginal lubrication less effective, with pain on penetration, an inevitable reaction of anxiety and a sense of inadequacy in the individuals involved. The vasocongestion of the male and female genitals, which takes place in the first phase of the sexual response and its alterations, have been known about since the very dawn of sexual medicine[66]. A slight difficulty in lubrication does not seem to interfere with sexual relations becaue the pain at the start of penetration wears off naturally as intercourse continues. When the occurrence of pain causes a state of anxiety that leads to avoiding sex, or when the pain persists, it can be dealt with by local gynecological pharmaceuticals, or else with interventions used in behavioral sexual medicine. Intense pain that does not go away by itself during intercourse, and that may also be present outside of an erotic encounter, is caused by situations of vaginal atrophy or dermatosis, interfering seriously in one's sex life. These conditions are frequent in old age, and lead to characteristic patterns that must be diagnosed by a gynecologist, and require specific pharmacological treatment. In the event of severe pain without an apparent physical cause, it is advisable to consult an expert in sexual medicine, because there are grounds for suspecting a negative approach to sexuality, as a consequence of a previous experience, of social considerations surrounding sexuality in elderly people, and one's own expectations over getting old. If the dyspareunia is caused by a reaction of hostility between the partners, then a specific therapeutic approach is needed.

The second change that is a direct result of aging presents more gradually over the years, and involves the intensity of orgasm. The physiological conditions of this phenomenon are clear. The orgasm, both in men and women, is a muscular response which, as such, feels the effects of the weakening of the pelvic floor, becoming less intense and less prolonged. With aging, all the muscles get weaker and lose their power to contract and their capacity for work, and so older people get tired more easily, and have less stamina even for activities that were habitual in the past. Body

---

66 Kaplan H.S., *The New Sex Therapy: Active Treatment of Sexual Dysfunctions*, Brunner/Mazel, New York, 1974.

mass and cardiorespiratory function influence muscular work in postmenopausal women, regardless of whether they take hormonal treatment[67], while the reduced responsiveness of muscle fibers to calcium reduces muscle power[68].

In women the pubococcygeal muscle, a branch of the levator ani muscle that surrounds the vaginal canal, is no exception to this rule, and its reduced force of contraction reduces pleasure. Naturally the basis of the orgasmic response is not solely organic but responds to previous experience, to desire and to health. In middle age it is especially influenced by negative attitudes toward oneself, and by sexual difficulties, but not by constant physical exercise, as happens by contrast in women who have not yet embarked on the menopausal transition[69].

To analyse the problem in a more precise way, we should note that, as well as being responsible for difficulties with orgasm, the loss of contractile force is at the origin of two conditions that are highly frequent among older women, namely urinary incontinence and a prolapsed uterus. The correlation between age and the weakening of the vaginal muscles seems to be independent of the number of pregnancies; the frequency of cystocele (prolapse of the bladder) or rectocele (prolapse of the anal canal) also increases after age 60, regardless of the number of vaginal births, and strikes around 40% of patients. Many women admit that a prolapse makes their sex life difficult, makes them feel less feminine, causes pelvic and lumbar pain, and causes embarrassent

67 Carvalho, Borghi-Silva, Dupontgand, et al., *Influence of menopausal status on the main contributors of muscle quality*, in "Climacteric", vol. 21, 2018, pp. 298–302.

68 Straight, Ades, Toth, *et al.*, *Age-related reduction in single muscle fiber calcium sensistivity is associated with decreased muscle power in men and women*, in "Exp Gerontol", vol. 102, 2018, pp. 84–92.

69 Ojanlatva, Mäkinen, Helenius, *et al.*, *Sexual activity and perceived health among Finnish middle-aged women*, in "Health and quality of life outcomes", vol. 4, 2006, p. 29.

due to the possibility of leaking urine during intercourse. Often the result is abstinence, especially in older women, and women without a stable partner[70].

A chronic condition such as asthma or a state of chronic pain, as with rheumatological illnesses, interferes with sexuality, especially in men. In these cases, abstinence from sex among a couple may reasonably be attributed to the compromised health of the man.

Imperfect sexuality

Human beings retain the ability to have sex throughout their lives, but a third of couples over age 65 become abstinent, and after 70 two thirds share this fate. With age, integrating intimacy, pleasure and eroticism in one's life becomes a source of deep gratification and makes the interaction between the partners more comfortable. A young man is used to regarding himself as autonomous as regards sexual performance, but, after age 60, a man and a woman have to be able to rely on each other to maintain a functional erotic relationship. This requires understanding, friendship and the ability to be open about one's needs, qualities which not all couples possess, however well they work together in day-to-day interaction. The effort is all about letting go of the idea of having control over a sexual perforance taking place in a predictable way, as was the case in the past. Although intercourse remains an integral part of the sexuality of couples of all ages, over time there is a need to be flexible in seeking pleasure, so that satisfaction can take place even when the erotic encounter is not automatically channeled towards penetration. Rather than lose sexual interaction due to aging, it is worth accepting

---

70 Panman, Wiegersma, Taisma, *et al.*, *Sexual function in older women with pelvic floor symptoms*, in "Br J Gen Pract", vol. 64, 2014, p. e144–149.

a certain reliance on mutual physical stimulation that improves excitement in women, and boosts the erection in the man. The response by the neurological and vascular systems also becomes less efficient; so, in order for sexuality to continue to be pleasurable and functional, more attention must be given to psychological, relational and sensual aspects in such a way as to compensate for physiological vulnerability. The route to survival is accepting that the sexual relationship is not always at its best, and giving greater value to erotic play and sensual stroking, both for women themselves and for help in boosting the genital erotic response. Around 5–15% of sexual encounters among couples over age 60 are dysfunctional; knowing this ought to make it easier for one to accept a playful and erotic sexuality, even when there is no penetration[71]. Shifting the emphasis onto erotic satisfaction rather than on performance improves the quality of the intimate relationship.

At times of difficulty, feelings of awkwardness prevent the partners from connecting emotionally. Even just exchanging brief glances, and simply looking toward each other in a way that may seem insignificant, is very valuable for maintaining intimacy. Turning to look toward the other, or instead looking the other way, even if this is due to personal suffering, and not out of any hostility, makes all the difference when it comes to safeguarding the relationship. Anxiety and uneasiness alter the emotional equilibrium, and often lead to involuntary errors of communication. Non-verbal signals are tenuous but powerful, and able to strongly influence the response by the person who receives them, even when they reflect even just a momentary denial or rejection. So it's important for couples who are facing reduced physical performance, and all the difficulties of aging, to manage to cultivate their relationship as it deserves, and to safeguard it in the event that a serious problem arises, with the

---

71 McCarthy, Metz, *The "good-enough sex" model: A case illustration*, in "Sex and Relat Ther", vol. 23, 2008, pp. 227–234.

awareness that communication may become difficult when it is associated with negative emotions such as concern over an illness, or a death[72].

Harmony, desire and celibacy

The frequency of sexual activity naturally diminishes with age, as Alfred Kinsey documented as far back as the 1950s, and it is affected by the inevitable changes brought by age. Despite the general trend toward less frequency, sexuality is a function of the vitality of the relationship, and of the harmony and erotic interest that have characterized the couple.

Aside from the physiology of aging, there are other factors in a relationship that contribute to inhibiting desire. Identifying an unattractive behavior in one's partner, and not succeeding in offsetting this with good qualities, is certainly a deterrent to desire, as sex therapists, Helen S. Kaplan first and foremost, know well. Often the loss of desire is a sign of a problem that can be resolved or not, depending on the interaction of many factors, such as love, that offset injured feelings, a commitment to keeping the relationship going, the support that comes from the wider family, etc etc.

Once the instinctive urgency of youth has passed, there is a need for a solid motivation that pushes toward a sexual relationship. When there is a constant lack of interest in an apparently gratifying relationship, one has to ask oneself what is wrong, and whether the failure lies in the ability to change and evolve, and to keep up with one's body as it changes.

As time passes, men and women become more and more reliant on romantic interaction and prolonged physical contact

---

72 Gottman J.M., Silver N., *The seven principles for making marriage work*, Harmony Books, New York, 2015.

in order to become aroused. Loving play does not begin in the bedroom; it begins with an act of kindness during the day, by showing an interest in the other person, by listening, and with a real desire to share. By the same token, desire is extinguished by unresolved arguments, criticism, unkind words, and all actions that are hurtful. In old age, anxiety and insecurity are the most frequent causes of difficulty in sexual behavior, and in order to resolve them it is crucial to be able to talk about oneself in an intimate way; it's unlikely that complications can be cleared up if the couple does not communicate, as is known to all those who are motivated in seeking a solution, and who therefore keep emotional dialogue alive and make the most of moments of tenderness. Instead of following the style of behavior that is no longer adequate, the couple that is aware of the new needs learns to take more time to allow sexual arousal to reach its peak. Paying attention to what constitutes pleasure and expanding the range of things to be done, like losing oneself in kisses and petting, can only make a relationship good and harmonious and result in an improvement in one's sex life. Specifically, women need to feel appreciated more than men; they respond with a higher emotional energy to affectionate support, and they find it difficult to put up with criticism. Negative interaction within the couple, often dictated by the limitations of daily life, places more of a burden on female satisfaction than other difficulties, personal or professional, that involve her alone. The positive side of the coin is that, despite the daily stresses, a devoted partner who is able to show his appreciation will always make his woman happy. Equally, it is not uncommon to see that, in many patients, sexual satisfaction goes hand in hand with the harmony of the relationship, a lot more than with personal motivation. In short, one could say that, for women, the quality of the relationship runs parallel to her quality of life.

One positive aspect that older women benefit from is that, with time, anxiety over having a perfect body becomes less acute, and acceptance of their real body, shaped by the events they have lived through, increases, and this allows them to see themselves as attractive. The quality of the relationship, intimacy, knowing each other, and significant communication are the key points of sexual satisfaction.

Some people choose not to go looking for sexual activity except within a stable relationship. This decison may be permanent, or it may reflect religious decisions, or one's philosophy of life; or it can be temporary, until such a time as a relationship becomes stabilized. The decision by people desiring a relationship not to engage in sex serves to develop an interpersonal intimacy that is not overly influenced by erotic activity. In other cases, it may be dictated by the need to focus on personal objectives that happen to be more important in that moment in time. Celibacy is a decision that in no way cancels out a woman's identity, or her sexual feelings; she remains aware of her identity and her reactions, even though she chooses not to take action. This situation is far from rare, when one considers that almost half of all women over 65 are widows. Working through grief over the death of one's partner is a difficult process, and it takes a long time. Equally, a lot of deep thought and feeling goes into accepting that the person who has passed on is part of one's life for all time, but, at the same time, one may manage to feel emotionally free to desire other relationships.

A real obstacle to sexuality for people who have been left by themselves in old age is the difficulty in finding a compatible partner for a relationship that can stimulate mutual desire.

The situation is different for women who, by their nature, or as a result of their previous experiences, have neither a desire nor an interest, and for whom old age has not led to any differences, and do not suffer from not having a romantic dimension in their life.

Further reading:

Levine S.B., *Sex is Not Simple*, Ohio Psychology Publishing Co., Columbus, 1988.

McCarthy B., McCarthy E., *Discovering Your Sexual Style*, Routledge, London, 2009.

Sager C.J., *Marriage Contracts and Couple Therapy*, Brunner/Mazel, New York, 1976.

Schiavi R.C., *Aging and Male Sexuality*, Cambridge Univ. Press, Cambridge, 1999.

J. Stephen Jones, *Overcoming Impotence*, Prometheus Books, New York, 2003

Levine S.B., *Sexual Life*, Plenum Press, New York, 1992.

Bancroft J, *Human Sexuality and Its Problems*, Churchill Livingstone, Edinburgh, 1989.

Kinsey A.C., Pomeroy W.B., Martin C.E., Gebhard P.H., *Sexual Behavior in the Human Female*, W.B. Saunders, Philadelphia, 1953.

Sherwin B.S., *The psychoendocrinology of aging and female sexuality: Annual review of sex research*, in "Society for the Scientific Study of Sex", 1991, pp. 181-198.

Bromberger, Schott, Kravitz, *Longitudinal change in reproductive hormones and depressive symptoms across the menopausal transition: Results from the study of women's health across the nation*, in "Arch Gen Psychiatry", 2010, pp. 598–607.

Freeman, Sammel, Boorman, Zhang, *Longitudinal pattern of depressive symptoms around natural menopause*, in "JAMA Psychiatry", vol. 71, pp. 36–43.

Hall K., *Reclaiming Your Sexual Self*, John Wiley & Sons, Hoboken, 2014.

Kaplan H.S., *Disorders of Sexual Desire*, Simon & Schuster, New York, 1979.

Foley S, Kope S.A. and Sugrue D.P., *Sex Matters for Women*, The Guilford Press, New York, 2012.

McCarthy B., McCarthy E., *Sexual Awareness*, Carroll & Graf Pub, New York, 1986.

CHAPTER 5

Dysfunctions in Sexual Behavior

Dysfunctions in sexual behavior present the same clinical picture, and the same causes, in the various different age groups: every dysfunction must, however, be viewed against the background of the single individual.

Age is certainly a vital factor in judging the adequacy of sexual behavior; the inability to reach orgasm for young women, and premature ejaculation for males, for example, are normal in early experiences, as is less frequent intercourse for elderly couples. It is also normal for the physiological changes of aging to interfere with lubrication and the erection, without there being intra-psychical or relational problems.

Unfortunately, the proven organic nature of the problem is no protection against the anxiety of an unpleasant experience, nor against a reaction of refusal, resulting from discouragement. Awareness is not enough to overcome the sorrow, the disappointment, and the sense of powerlessness over something that seems impossible to resolve. In some instances, the reaction of acute anxiety may be so predominant as to conceal an organic cause. A condition cannot be allowed to remain hidden beneath the weight of emotions; it has to be recognised and treated.

The hormonal changes of menopause reduce the elasticity of the vagina and the production of lubricating mucous, penetration becomes difficult and painful, if not impossible, and one's sex life becomes affected by this. While the negative role of vulvovaginal atrophy is easy to recognise, conditions affecting the pelvic floor, genital prolapse, and urinary incontinence are no less harmful.

Genital prolapse occurs when organs contained in the pelvis, such as the bladder and the uterus, slip down from their position and form a protuberance inside the vagina. This situation is caused by the fact the levator ani loses strength due to traumatic births, or due to aging. The lowering may be so pronounced that the uterus reaches the vulva, and protrudes from the body.

Urinary incontinence is the result of loss of voluntary control in urination. When one sneezes, coughs or laughs suddenly, the body passes water in a strong jet, owing to the increase in abdominal pressure; in other cases there is a very slight but constant drip.

Urinary incontinence is an independent condition, often of neurological origin, but involuntary leakage is also a symptom of a prolapse, because the lowering of the uterus changes the position of the bladder, and alters the function of the sphincters. Although they are two different conditions, a prolapse and incontinence both lead to urine leakage during intercourse, with an emotional response ranging from embarrassment to feelings of inadequacy, and may involve a deterioration of one's body image.

In terms of common social conditioning, involuntarily passing water in public is an awful and highly embarrassing situation, just as when it happens in moments of intimacy. Many women feel inadequate as sexual partners, and do not manage to confide in their partner, preferring instead to give up having a sex life. The fear of such a mortifying event happening leads to embarrassment, shame, and the build-up of anxiety, which worsen the quality of life more than is warranted by the episode in itself.

The pain on penetration caused by atrophy, the embarrassment over the altered aesthetic appearance of the protrusion of the uterus, and anxiety over the potential passing of water all place a burden on the sexual relationship even in long-standing couples. In these cases, knowing one can count on the support of one's lifelong companion is already part of the solution. Knowing the other person well means it becomes possible to find simple and effective solutions, like going to the bathroom immediately before intercourse, laying an absorbent coverlet on the bed, or using plenty of lubricant, also on the penis… In the right situation, one can also take away any tension by having a laugh about it!

When intimacy is maintained and the relationship is emotionally gratifying, physical contact in the form of stroking and hugs reawakens epidermic pleasure, and facilitates sexuality.

However, not all couples who grow old together are so lucky. For those who share lifelong habits (such as looking after the family), but who no longer have a deep understanding, it is difficult to show complicity over the effects of illness. It is easier to retreat and avoid erotic interactions which could trigger tensions. Understandably, not feeling attractive makes it embarrassing to be naked, and dispels erotic thoughts and feelings.

Indeed, there is a complex relationship between one's emotional state, advanced age, and the impoverishment of one's sex life. Age always correlates with frequency, but when one starts to perceive anxiety over one's aesthetic appearance, this appearance becomes the biggest single determining factor of sexuality, even in older women[73].

A reaction of rejection of sexual intimacy that suffers a lot from the aesthetic component is seen in women who have had an operation for breast cancer. There are many causes for the emotional and relational difficulties of these patients, from the impact on one's mood of the diagnosis of a life-threatening illness, to the secondary effects of powerful drugs that alter many metabolic functions, including pronounced hormonal alterations. As the years go by, when this is a thing of the past, and the woman has completely recovered, there remains the difficulty of accepting the aesthetics of the breast that has been operated on. The image of one's injured body is so powerful that women who choose reconstruction do not seem much more satisfied than those who remain with the signs of the operation[74]. The scar recalls the illness, and makes a woman feel less feminine. Almost all patients

---

73 Handelzalts, Yaakobi, Levy *et alii*, *The impact of genital self-image on sexual function in women with pelvic floor disorders,* in "Eur J Obstet Gyn Repr Biol", vol. 211, 2017, pp. 164–168.

74 Hummel, Hahn, van Lankveld *et alii*, *Factors associated with specific diagnostic and statistical manual of mental disorders, fourth edition sexual dysfunctions in breast cancer survivors: A study of patients and their partners,* in "J Sex Med", vol. 14, pp. 1248–1259.

feel the need to exclude it from their romantic moments, they don't show it and don't allow it to be stroked.

Those who do not resume their sex life even after recovery, and after regaining a certain serenity, blame this on the loss of physical intimacy, many of the women who become sexually active again have never again shown themselves completely naked, so as not to lose their sense of their own femininity, while patients who are not in a stable relationship, and who would like to begin a romantic relationship are especially anxious over the way the scar may be perceived; they fear that it may be a deterrent, they feel fragile and are convinced that they will not be accepted by a possible partner[75].

Embarrassment and shame are reactions that impoverish the sex life of many female patients who have suffered organic damage, but they don't always lead to total abstinence from sex. When one's sex life is suspended, there are multiple causes, including the loss of motivation and relationship factors, such as a lack of support from one's partner; by contrast, women with modest symptoms stay active if they can count on a good erotic understanding, and if they have had a gratifying life in the past. Indeed, among women in a stable relationship who have urinary incontinence, the oldest prefer to avoid sex, but most continue to have sex, although they recognise certain limitations. Only 5% report that they no longer have sexual relations[76].

The man contributes to the couple's sex life with his desire and his capabilities, but age changes also affect him. After age 60, men may develop secondary dysfunctions as a result of common

---

75 Hummel, van Lankveld, Oldenburg *et alii*, *Efficacy of internet-based cognitive behavioral therapy in improving sexual functioning of breast cancer survivors: Results of a randomized controlled trial*, in "J Clin Oncol", vol. 35, 2017, pp. 1328–1340.

76 Visser, de Book, Berger, *et alii*, *Impact of urinary incontinence on sexual functioning in community-dwelling older women*, in "J Sex Med", vol. 11, 2014, pp. 1757–1765.

organic conditions such as diabetes, hypertension and cardiovascular illnesses; moreover, some very well-used drugs such as antidepressants, anti-hypertensives, diuretics, and medication for the cardiovascular system may cause or worsen a dysfunction[77]. The most common one involves the erection, which tends to be achieved more slowly, or which is not 100% complete, or which may diminish during intercourse; understandably, erectile dysfunction undermines the sex life of a couple that is already affected by the woman's own difficulties. The dual fragility makes each partner more understanding toward the other, but it doubles the very real difficulties in making love, and the problem of anxiety which the man also develops.

In cases where the low level of intimacy makes it hard to talk to each other about what makes each one suffer, misunderstandings and moodiness can have a damaging effect and lead to abstinence, whereas when there is good harmony, it becomes possible to solve dysfunctions, and indeed many couples do not give up sex, despite the general worsening.

For man, prostate cancer is a mirror of breast cancer. This affects an organ that is a symbol of sexuality. Erectile difficulty affects up to 100% of men after the operation, but anxiety and denial are so strong that fewer than 50% of couples are interested in rehabilitation[78].

Sexuality is, by definition, a shared activity, and it is affected by the state of health, physical capabilities, and the interest of both partners; in couples that have been together for many years, it is the result of the compromise between the expectations and preferences of each of the two, a compromise that is set to change as a situation gradually changes, as happens when one grows old.

---

77 Rew, Heidelbaugh, *Erectile dysfunction*, in "Am Fam Physician", vol. 94, 2016, pp. 820–827.

78 McCullogh, *Prevention and management of erectile dysfunction following radical prostatectomy*, in "Urol Clin North Am", vol. 28, 2001, pp. 613–627.

In general, people of this age do not want to see changes in their partner, say they are satisfied, and have a low rate of divorce. However, there is some friction also in the case of these women, and the bone of contention seems to lie in poor communication, especially regarding intimacy.

It is vital to be able to express one's true feelings, but after a certain age men and women tend to confide more easily in a friend than with their partner, so that they can get reassurance without bringing discontent into the home. This probably happens because many older people do everything they can to prevent open conflict, in order to maintain a serene atmosphere.

Sexual rehabilitation

Conditions like genital atrophy, urinary incontinence and uterine prolapse can be treated with interventions that are part of the regular armamentarium of gynecology. This, depending on pathology and severity, uses oral and topical medications, rehabilitation physiotherapy, and surgical procedures.

Sexual dysfunctions originating from these conditions cannot always be resolved with the amelioration of the organic function, but they can be effectively dealt with by means of interventions specific to behavioral sex therapy, like Kegel exercises, vaginal cones, and vaginal dilators.

Kegel exercises consist of voluntary and rhythmic contractions of the pubococcygeal muscles that the patient performs daily, while vaginal cones of increasing weight are progressively inserted into the vagina to ameliorate its contracting strength.

Vaginal dilators are a series of small cylinders of increasing size that the patient uses privately. They gently act on the vaginal walls, ameliorating their elasticity, and lessening the pressure pain at penetration.

Nevertheless, these interventions may still be to no avail if there is not enough intimacy to carry them out. Unfortunately, when making love becomes difficult, even the simplest signs of affection tend to become few and far between. Without kissing, holding, and caressing, the connection with the other's body is lost, even though affection may remain unchanged. To help couples regain an intimacy with their partner's body, we apply sex therapy interventions, called sensate focus exercises.

In the course of therapy, partners are guided to gradually rebuild their physical closeness by mutually caressing each other's bodies. At the beginning of therapy, genitals are excluded, to avoid anxiety reactions and, for the same reason, exposing one's body completely naked is also avoided, which is reassuring for highly sensitive patients, as in the case of women who have had a mastectomy. For all, and mostly for oncology patients, the exercises performed together with one's partner are crucial for rebuilding the couple's harmony.

Body image is a complex projection of physical appearance and seduction, which oncology patients can regain also with the help of a group psychotherapy program[79]. Thanks to the fact that pleasurable feelings gradually return, uneasiness stemming from the disease can be overcome, desire is revived, and sexual relations become possible again.

Men who have undergone surgery for prostate cancer, a very frequent event in men in their 60s and 70s, can also benefit from sensate focus exercises. The inevitable surgical procedures are responsible for erectile difficulties that can be managed with the use of pharmacological or physical prosthesis.

The former are used when there is neurological damage, but the corpora cavernosa tissues remain healthy and capable of producing an erection with the increase of blood flow.

---

79 Esplen, Wong, Warner *et alii*, *Restoring body image after cancer (reBIC): results of a randomized controlled trial*, in "J Clin. Oncol.", vol. 36, 2018, pp. 749–756.

Physical prosthetics are required, on the other hand, when the erectile tissues suffer metabolic damage, and are no longer capable of producing an erection.

The various different interventions are effective in resolving organic damage, but do not extend to emotional problems, and do not solve relational or sexual discomfort. Clinical experience tells us that, in these patients too, sensate focus exercises promote a connection of pleasure and intimacy while removing anxiety, using the same mechanisms that are effective for any other couple affected by an organic condition.

Medications for menopause

Hormonal treatment for menopause, usually called replacement therapy (HRT), consists of formulations made of estrogens, or an association of estrogens and progestin. It is likely that no other subject in the field of gynecology is as controversial as prescribing hormones during menopause, as it presents side effects that cannot be overlooked, despite its undeniable benefits. Of these, it is not yet clear what correlation exists between HRT and the incidence of cancer in the reproductive organs that was first suspected about twenty years ago. Since then, new studies and observational data have allowed a more balanced evaluation of hormone metabolic action, while the ratio between oncology risk and amelioration of quality of life is considered favorable when therapy begins at the same time as the onset of menopause, and is carried out for about 3–5 years[80].

HRT is the most effective treatment to reduce vasomotor symptoms (hot flashes), to combat vaginal atrophy, and to prevent the

---

80 Ward, Deneris, *An update on menopause management*, in "J Midwifery Womens Health", vol. 63, 2018, pp. 1–10.

loss of bone tissue. The risks associated with treatment include worsening of cardiovascular function, coagulation, and cognition, and these vary depending on factors such as the type of drug, its duration and means of administration, and timing, meaning the time interval between the last menstrual cycle and when it is first taken. These different methods and conditions explain why the choice between different pharmaceutical preparations has to be made by the attending physician, in accordance with the clinical history of each patient. As of today, it seems generally accepted that the treatment has a more favorable profile, in terms of effectiveness and lower metabolic risk, when it is first taken before age 60, or within less than ten years from the last menstrual cycle.

Women who are over 60, or at more than ten years from their last menses, are at higher risk of developing a cardiovascular pathology, or thromboembolism, or a worsening of their cognitive functions.

HRT comes in two formulations: one contains only estrogens, and the other combines estrogens and progestin; the choice between the two must be made according to exact rules to limit possible unfavorable side effects. The risk of breast cancer when taking just estrogens is small, but the increase of uterine cancer is well documented, with percentages that depend on the dosage and the duration of treatment. The association of estrogens and progestins is protective for the endometrium, as it keeps the risk of hyperplasia or uterine cancer at the same level as untreated women, but taking them for more than five years increases the incidence of breast cancer.

New SERM substances (selective ER modulators) represent an alternative to the use of progestin, as they prevent endometrial hyperplasia[81] and offer protection against uterine cancer, with-

---

81 Increase in the mucous tissue of the uterus.

out increasing the risk of breast cancer. Some observational data suggest a possible but rare increase of ovarian cancer following prolonged use of HRT. However, these findings are not yet confirmed.

Treatment can proceed in oral, transvaginal, or transdermal fashion. These different types of administering the therapy have different impacts in terms of their side effects.

Medications taken orally are metabolized by the liver before they can be absorbed. During this hepatic stage, they stimulate the production of substances facilitating blood coagulation and increasing the risk of thrombosis; at the same time, they raise the blood concentration of lipoprotein, triglycerides, and reactive C protein, thus creating an unfavorable state for the cardiovascular system.

Transdermal preparations have fewer side effects, as they do not need the initial hepatic phase in order to be absorbed; in addition, they use a smaller amount of active substance to maintain stable concentrations, because they enter the bloodstream directly, through the skin. They are preferred in women with a higher risk of cardiovascular pathologies, or women who are older[82].

Taking hormone therapy is usually contraindicated in patients with irregular bleedings, hepatic pathology, or a predisposition to breast or uterine cancers, or to cardiovascular, metabolic or thromboembolic conditions; furthermore, prudence is necessary in treating patients with migraine, uterine myomas, or endometriosis as these conditions may worsen under the influence of the prescribed hormones.

---

82 Kopper, Gudeman, Thompson, *Transdermal hormone therapy in postmeno-pausal women: A review of metabolic effects and drug delivery technologies*, in "Drug Design, Development and Therapy", vol. 2, 2009, pp. 193–202.

It must be underlined that, even in healthy patients, HRT treatment involves a higher risk of deep venous thrombosis or hepatic and circulatory pathologies, and that the motivation for treatment must always be discussed and clarified with one's physician.

The effects of hormone replacement therapy

Vasomotor symptoms are the symptoms that see an absolute improvement with hormone treatment; a beneficial side effect of the reduction of hot flashes and night sweats is the improvement of sleep patterns, thanks to the reduction of broken nights.

HRT helps to maintain balance when standing and walking, thanks to the fact that it combats the loss of bone tissue and osteoporosis; moreover, it offers a potential benefit for the reduction of broken bones, despite the fact it has to be accompanied by a diet designed to insure an intake of calcium and vitamin D and adequate physical exercise. The drug acts on the biomechanical structure of joints, making sure they continue to function properly, and gives protection against osteoarthritis (better known as arthrosis), by means of a mechanism that is not yet clear. A small but growing number of studies suggests that hormone therapy helps to preserve good muscle function, maintaining muscle mass, its ability to contract, and connective tissue; it also seems that it improves functional recovery after a trauma when it is associated with appropriate physical exercises.

We know that the deprivation of estrogens increases the deposit of abdominal fat, alterations in the lipid profile and resistence to insulin which, in turn, facilitates diabetes; hormone therapy provides protection against these metabolic effects, and it reduces the increase in abdominal fat and in the body mass index, which reflect the lipid profile; it also moderately reduces the incidence of colon cancer, but it does not seem to have any beneficial effect on cardiocirculatory pathologies. A negative action is seen on the function of the liver and of the gallbladder, especially for oral preparations, which increase the production of bile and the risk of calculus. One thing to always be borne in mind is the rise in thromboembolic events, which represent a serious risk to health, and which can strike women of all ages.

The effects of HRT on mood and cognitive function are not thoroughly understood, but they seem mildly positive, while the effect on memory seems neutral. Regarding Alzheimer's, it seems that the therapy is protective if begun soon, and that it increases the risk of this disease if started too late after the last menstrual cycle; it is certain that these effects also depend largely on the cognitive state of the patient before treatment.

The metabolic effects seem to depend on the time it is taken: the metabolic profile is more favorable the nearer to the onset of menopause it is started. The risk/benefit ratio on cognitive function is less favorable when it is taken late, regardless of how it is administered. In any event, all these findings are preliminary, and need to be confirmed by further studies[83].

Prolonged use, lasting five or more years, maintains control of vasomotor symptoms and slows down the incidence of osteoporosis; this form of treatment should be provided in the case of serious symptoms that continue over time, and that do not respond to other treatments. The benefits are not negligible, because there is a 50% chance that hot flashes will present again, while osteoporosis progresses and becomes ever more serious, because it is affected by the mechanisms of aging and not only of the changes of menopause. Naturally, the advisability of prolonged use must be assessed for each patien in light of their metabolic state, and the side effects of the drug.

Women over age 65 who are otherwise healthy, who do not have a profile of increased risk of liver or citculatory conditions, and who decide to continue to take hormones have a statistically significant lower number of fractures, and manage to maintain

---

83 Lewis, Wellons, *Menopausal hormone therapy for primary prevention of chronic disease*, in "JAMA", vol. 12, 2017, pp. 2187–2189.

a good level of mobility, but they must be aware that they may suffer episodes of thromboembolism or dementia. If the patient requests this, and if her attending doctor believes that, under careful supervision, the benefits outweigh the risks, it may be acceptable to continue to take hormones in the lowest possible dose, and not interrupt this on the basis of age alone [84]

Hormone therapy and prevention of chronic illnesses

Some chronic conditions such as cardiocirculatory pathologies, diabetes, dementia, some tumors, and osteoporosis, which are found with very high frequency in post-menopause, are the result of hormonal changes (and not just aging mechanisms) and can only partially be prevented. In light of the benefits that hormone therapy may offer, the idea came into being of using it not as a treatment but for the purposes of prevention in patients who show no sign of illness. If a drug is used for prevention, its side effects must be considered very carefully, using a very different level of caution from that required for controlling symptoms already present, and for which there is a specific indication. Despite the initially favorable suggestions, so far the use of HRT is not recommended for the primary prevention of chronic diseases owing to its side effects, which worsen the risk/benefit ratio, both in patients with an intact uterus and in patients who have had theirs removed[85].

---

84 North American Menopause Society, The North American Menopause Society statement on continuing use of systemic hormone therapy after age 65, in "Menopause", vol. 22, 2015, p. 693.

85 Jin, *Hormone therapy for primary prevention of chronic conditions in postmenopausal women*, in "JAMA", vol. 12, 2017, p. 2265.

Prescribing hormones for prevention is not indicated in healthy women, while it is indicated for women who are in situations of particular fragility due to early menopause, both natural and surgically induced.

Maintaining well-being in early menopause

When menopause presents early, its effects are particularly devastating to health and quality of life. Metabolic damage appears and, unless timely action is taken, it becomes worse as time goes by, eventually creating health conditions that are not compatible with the age of the patient.

So-called *premature ovarian failure* (POF) is the term used when a woman below age 40 loses menstruations and has menopausal-type hormonal values. It strikes around 1% of women of fertile age. The diagnosis is devastating for a young woman who finds herself having to face a state of untimely menopause, and it is even more painful for women who have not had children, because it is extremely unlikely that these patients can have a pregnancy. The condition may be associated with autoimmune illnesses or chromosomal anomalies, but its cause remains unknown in 90% of cases[86].

We talk of *early menopause* when the cessation of menstrual cycles occurs between the ages of 40 and 45, around 10 years before the average age. The event can come about through natural causes, often unexplained, and it strikes around 5% of women in this age group[87]. One known cause could be ovarian damage as a result of oncology treatments, especially for breast cancer, which suppress the production of steroid hormones and menstruations.

---

86 Kovanci, Schutt, *Premature ovarian failure: clinical presentation and treatment*, in "Obstet Gynecol Clin North Am"», vol. 42, 2015, pp. 153–216.

87 Shuster, Rhodes, Gostout *et alii*, *Premature menopause or early menopause: Long-term health consequences*, in "Maturitas", vol. 65, 2010, pp. 161–166.

In most cases, however, early menopause is the result of the surgical removal of the ovaries for a benign condition, such as fibromas and cysts, affecting the uterus or the ovaries themselves. Even women who have kept their ovaries in the course of a hysterectomy run the risk of having an early menopause, because the anatomical changes linked to the operation alter the blood flow to the pelvis; this condition is associated with early aging of the adnexa, which becomes evident just six months after the operation.

The surgical removal of the ovaries in women of fertile age is a rare but dramatic event, resulting in the sudden loss of all the steroids that they produce: estrogens, progesterone and testosterone. The negative effects are much more dramatic than those seen with natural menopause or with early menopause, where hormone production ceases gradually, and the organism has a certain amount of time to adapt to a new climate.

Regardless of what causes early menopause, health suffers from the pathologies that result from it. Women who enter menopause before their time have to live in a state of estrogen deprivation a lot longer than other women of the same age, and deal with the consequences of it, heightened by the early age of onset. These patients have an increased risk of neurological disease, cardiocirculatory illness, and a state of infertility. Often present are signs of depression, anxiety, or psychiatric pathologies that are a response to the feeling of not being able to live adequately.

Unless there are important contraindications, it is a good idea to promptly prescribe hormone replacement therapy to combat conditions that could have devastating effects on health and quality of life.

Other pharmacological and non-pharmacological interventions

Vulvovaginal atrophy

Estrogen-based and progesterone-based parenteral pharmacological regimes are not the only possible treatments for the symptoms of menopause. Other hormone preparations are used with the principle that, in order to treat an organ, it is not necessary to treat the whole organism. This can be achieved with preparations based on estrogens alone. These are very different than HRT, because they are available in the form of creams or vaginal suppositories for local application.

The latter are regarded as the best form of treatment for vulvovaginal atrophy, and prove to be effective against pain during intercourse, burning, and dryness. Vulvovaginal atrophy is also called "genitourinary syndrome", especially by American writers, in acknowledgement of the fact that in serious cases it causes alterations of the urinary function.

The atrophic pattern is a result of the reduction of estrogen occurring in natural menopause and in other pathologies. The alteration of the genital tissues consists in reduced blood flow, reduced elasticity, and the thinning of the epithelium, all factors that contribute to pain in intercourse, with overlapping mechanisms that increase each other: the reduced elasticity makes penetration difficult, and the reduced epithelium does not produce enough lubricating mucous. By means of a series of biochemical reactions, the thinning of the mucosa alters vaginal pH, and makes the environment more susceptible to inflammation, which can be difficult to treat, for the very reason that the natural factors of protection are lost. The use of estrogens in the form of local preparations combats these changes effectively, insofar as it helps vaginal epithelium to regain its integrity and its ability to function; indeed, thanks to the treatment, they increase the number of cells in the superficial layer, flora and pH values are restored, and vaginal lubrication is improved.

Since the condition of atrophy tends to return, and to get worse, local preparations in low doses can be used for long periods of time, as long as patients are checked regularly; unfortunately, the risk cannot yet completely excluded that local treatment may increase the risk of cancer of the endometrium (although, for example, using it for a period of two years seems safe).

Giving local estrogens is not recommended in women with previous tumors, with risk factors for tumors sensitive to estrogen, or with coagulation problems. Local treatments based on lubricants or moisturizers that improve vaginal dryness are one possible alternative.

In the presence of situations that are not particularly serious, the first choice consists of one or more cycles of non-hormonal preparations such as gels and creams, with differing effects that can also be used in association with each other. As well as moisturizing and lubricating creams and gels, there are other options for restructuring vaginal epithelium; these include new non-hormonal oral drugs (like Ospemiphene), behavioral sex therapy interventions, and laser applications[88].

An alternative for patients who cannot take hormones, and whose condition does not improve with the use of lubricants and moisturizers, involves behavioral interventions such as exercises to relax the pelvic floor, and using vaginal dilators. The exercises are performed by the patient in the privacy of her own home, and, when possible, with the participation of her partner, but they have to be guided by an experienced doctor.

One tool able to alleviate dryness and burning is the CO_2 Laser for micro ablation, which offers an alternative to estrogen treatment for women with dyspareunia. When a combination of local estrogens and laser applications is given, one achieves a result that is so effective that the results are maintained for over 20

---

88 Sousa, Peate, Jarvis *et alii*, *A clinical guide to the management of genitourinary symptoms in breast cancer survivors on endocrine therapy*, in "Ther Adv Med Oncol.", vol. 9, 2017, pp. 269–285.

weeks[89]. The use of the CO2 Laser has proved especially useful in women who have suffered from breast cancer. Being able to rely on the effectiveness of a well tolerated treatment that has no side effects is vital for treating patients with serious dyspareunia, and who, owing to their primary condition, cannot proceed with hormone treatment.

All the preparations and all the interventions presented have a certain effectiveness in improving the state of atrophy and slowing down the further changes of the menopause and of aging, but they cannot reconstruct tissue, and so it is important that women are informed in time regarding manifestations of and possible remedies for vaginal atrophy. Choosing the treatment depends on the seriousness of the symptoms, on the increased risk of oncological conditions, and personal preferences.

Vasomotor symptoms

The most effective treatment against vasomotor symptoms is hormone treatment. Unfortunately, however, it is not suitable for all patients, owing to its metabolic effects, and the possible rise in oncological risk. In view of the metabolic profile of hormone treatment, it is reasonable to resort to effective but non-pharmacological interventions as the first choice of form of treatment, ones which, at the same time, can be suited to patients for whom HRT is contraindicated.

The psychoeducational approach is based on relaxation techniques involving either breathing or the muscles, or else on behavioral strategies. The effectiveness of relaxation techniques ranges from moderate to highly significant, with a reduction of

---

89 Cruz, Steiner, Pompei *et alii*, *Randomized, double-blind, placebo-controlled clinical trial for evaluating the efficacy of fractional CO2 laser compared with topical estriol in the treatment of vaginal atrophy in postmenopausal women*, in "Menopause", vol. 25, 2018, pp. 21–28.

symptoms that can be as much as 73%, with results maintained for more than six months. The explanation for this variability is the influence played by the close patient-doctor relationship on satisfaction with the treatment, and also the presence of a recognisable placebo effect, able to reduce vasomotor symptoms by 30% without active interventions; however, the data is still insufficient to be able to say whether all these techniques are more effective than the placebo, or than no intervention, in reducing the number and seriousness of hot flashes over a 24-hour period.

Among possible treatments for those who prefer to avoid taking hormones, acupuncture seems to have a moderately positive effect on the frequency of vasomotor episodes, but most of all on their seriousness, without adverse effects. A further alternative is represented by physical exercise and yoga, but, in these cases too, the benefits in reducing hot flashes seem never more than modest.

Food, extracts and dietary supplements that contain high levels of phytoestrogens (soya isoflavones) can mildly alleviate the frequency and seriousness of vasomotor symptoms, without effects on the endometrium or vagina. *Cimicifuga racemosa*[90], traditionally used by Native Americans, seems to represent a further, reasonable alternative, but in this case too the results have only a minimum level of significance[91].

In conclusion, the effectiveness of alternative treatments is very modest, at least in terms of statistical rigor, but this must not discourage patients from trying out whatever does not have adverse effects, and from choosing the most effective treatment for them.

When HRT is unsuitable, undesired, or not tolerated, the best choice for combating vasomotor symptoms of a certain seriousness is represented by treatment using new-generation antidepressants. The symptoms are reduced by up to 70% within 6–12 weeks, and, compared with their real effectiveness, these

---

90 Plant with anti-inflammatory and rebalancing properties.
91 Carroll, Lisenby, Carter, *Critical appraisal of paroxetine for the treatment of vasomotor symptoms*, in "Int J Womens Health", vol. 7, 2015, pp. 615–624.

drugs have only minimal side effects, restricted to constipation and nausea, which disappear within the first week. The treatment begins at the lowest possible dose, which, if necessary, can be gradually increased.

Diet

Appetite, and the ritual nature of mealtimes, are the product of psychological and social motivations, and also of the need to keep biological functions active. Food with a high protein content, consumed together with fruit, vegetables and legumes, has a beneficial effect on female fertility. Specifically, higher consumption of pasta, wholemeal bread and cereals protects against the onset of early menopause, which does not happen with the consumption of animal proteins. The same protective effect is achieved by having a calcium intake, from milk and dairy products, such as yogurt and cheese (both fresh and mature), especially when associated with vitamin D.

Biological needs regulate food intake, the expenditure of energy for metabolic functions, and muscular work, by means of various mechanisms. Fluctuations in estrogens control one's food intake, and the deposit of adipose tissue in all phases of a woman's life. Evident demonstrations are an increase in abdominal fat in menopause, and a preference for high-calorie sweets, which increases during the menstrual cycle. Estrogen action can explain gender differences when it comes to disturbances of eating habits, such as anorexia, and bulimia (as well as obesity), both of which are more frequent in women than in men.

As happens in the case of many mammals that have a prolonged luteal phase[92] (sheep, monkeys and hamsters), the female human reduces food intake at the time of ovulation, when

---

92 Phase of around 14 days, from ovulation to the arrival of menstruation.

concentrations of estrogens are at their peak. But that is not all. Their fluctuations influence eating habits, calorie intake, and variations in appetite during the menopausal transition, and in the post-menopause phase.

In the years of transition, one sees a gradual increase in appetite, and the desire to eat, and more frequent snacks, as well as a reduction in the amount of food ingested, and consequently a reduction of proteins, fats and carbohydrates. Despite the lower intake of calories, fat mass increases in body composition, probably due to the lower expenditure of energy caused by an increasingly sedentary lifestyle. When the transition is over and menopause stabilizes, eating habits change again. In these years, there tends to be a rise in the consumption of proteins and carbohydrates, and especially of fatty meals, although many women voluntarily choose a rigorous diet to avoid gaining weight.

Obesity increases in post-menopausal women, showing that reduced concentrations of estrogen lead to an accumulation of body fat; with the same mechanism, replacement therapy reconstructs estrogen levels and combats the build-up of fat, although it is unclear whether it acts by means of a lower food intake or with direct action on adipose tissue[93].

Metabolic effects of different foods

The estrogen climate in women of fertile age protects them from metabolic syndrome, an advantage that disappears in menopause, when abdominal fat starts to be deposited. Especially in the West, the great availability of high-calorie and appetising foods invites consumption that is far above metabolic needs and the need for energy, with an inevitable increase in

---

93 Butera, *Estradiol and the control of food intake*, in "Physiol Behav", vol. 99, 2010, pp. 175–180.

the percentage of obesity, in which women in menopause are a particularly easy target, due to both the absence of estrogens and their sedentary lifestyle[94].

Taking food in its various components plays a part in the metabolic mechanisms of menopause with an effect that has repercussions on organs and functions. An intake of fruit and vegetables brings vitamins, minerals and fibers, which combat cardiocirculatory disease, satisfy the appetite, and protect against consuming foods with a higher calorie content. Consuming abundant fruit and vegetables continually over a period of 8 years protects against obesity, but this result is influenced by physical activity and body weight at the start of the menopausal transition. Fruit and vegetables presumably protect against an increase in weight thanks to their calcium, potassium and magnesium content, the antioxidant and anti-inflammatory properties of polyphenols, and the presence of water and fiber, which make one feel full.

In the last few decades, the use of prepared foods has spread. These have a content of fat, sugar and especially salt that is higher than freshly-made meals. The excessive intake of sodium and lipids represents a risk factor for atherosclerosis and for coronary disease, especially for women with abdominal obesity and hypertension, or who were overweight even before age 65, and who have a high probability of falling ill. By contrast, a diet that is low in sodium reduces the damage and protects against metabolic illnesses, ie hypercholesterolemia, diabetes and hypertension, which lie at the root of cardiocirculatory pathologies.

The Mediterranean diet gained popularity in the 1960s, when it was noted that local populations, especially the Italians and Greeks, had a lower death rate from cardiovascular incidents compared to northern Europe and North America. Sticking to a diet that comprises oil, legumes, cereals, flour, fruit, vegetables, fish

---

94 Rivera, Stincic, *Estradiol and the control of feeding behavior*, in "Steroids", vol. 133, 2017, pp. 44–52.

and modest amounts of wine, meat, milk and dairy products is effective in reducing cholesterol and lipoproteins[95].

When combined with physical activity and maintaining body weight, a diet rich in antioxidants and polyphenols, but low on red meat and alcohol, and that includes fruit, vegetables, olive oil and fiber, as in the Mediterranean diet, seems able to give metabolic protection that can reduce the incidence of breast cancer.

Breast cancer, which is increasingly frequent in Western women, recognises risk factors linked to lifestyle such as diet, smoking, obesity and a sedentary lifestyle, which create a state of inflammation located in breast tissue, together with environmental causes and genetic mutations which, in the last few decades, seem to have increased their power to act[96].

Despite the fact that alcohol is often regarded as harmful to health, regular consumption without excesses does not alter the body weight or metabolism of healthy post-menopausal women[97].

Changes in everyday behavior linked to age (lower food intake, less physical movement, and reduced hormone levels) help to reduce muscle mass and its contractile force. It is worrying to think that the loss of muscle mass begins at age 50 and continues throughout one's life. At age 80, one's muscles have reduced by around 40% of their level at their peak, at age 20. This condition alters one's posture, increases the frequency of falls and broken bones, and impacts the quality of life and survival.

95 Rees, Jartley, Flowers *et alii*, *"Mediterranean" dietary pattern for the primary prevention of cardiovascular disease*, in "Cochrane Database of Systematic Reviews", vol. 12, 2013.

96 Shapira, *The potential contribution of dietary factors to breast cancer prevention*, in "European Journal of Cancer Prevention", vol. 26, 2017, pp. 385–395.

97 Wang, Lee, Manson *et alii*, *Alcohol consumption, weight gain, and risk of becoming overweight in middle-aged and older women*, in "Arch Intern Med", vol. 170, 2010, pp. 453–461.

The process is inevitable, but some things can be done to lessen it. An adequate diet is vitally important to maintain muscle mass and prevent sarcopenia, ie the reduction of mass that is seen in elderly people, especially when they follow imbalanced diets. A diet with a low protein content is associated with a greater presence of body fat, poor function of the upper and lower limbs, and a loss of physical capablities. This is a danger because it also reduces balance when standing erect and walking, it causes falls, and, not infrequently, broken bones. It causes debilitation of the body, but cognitive functions are unchanged. A protein-rich diet can improve a state of sarcopenia that is already present, even in people who are very old, increasing muscle strength and physical performance[98].

The consumption of proteins has a positive effect on the skeleton, it is directly associated with bone density in the neck of the femur, the trochanter and the vertebras, especially in women who have a low calcium intake, and it represents a factor that combats osteoporosis. Indeed, proteins and calcium are the biggest components of bone tissue; they play an active part in bone metabolism and depend on each other. It seems that a higher intake of proteins encourages the absorption of calcium, improving bone density. By contrast, a diet low in proteins is associated with a thinning of the structure of the neck of the femur in women over age 50.

These observations underline once again the importance of an adequate diet to reduce as much as possible the loss of bone tissue with aging, especially because improving protein intake is not enough to restore bone density in the short term.

The beneficial effect that a diet containing proteins and calcium has on bone health maintains density, slows down the loss of tissue, and reduces the risk of fractured bones. Resistence to traumas is an essential feature of bones, involving all the components:

---

98 Gregorio, Brindisi, Kleppinger, *Adequate dietary protein is associated with better physical performance among post-menopausal women 60-90 years*, in "J Nutr Health Aging", vol.18, 2014; pp. 155–160.

cell renewal, the outer part (cortical bone), and the internal rabecular bone.

Milk seems to be the foodstuff most associated with strength and maintaining the structure of peripheral bones (the limbs), because it provides protein and calcium at the same time; indeed, the amount of milk consumed is inversely proportional to the frequency of pelvic fractures.

Strength, the microstructure of bones, and protein and calcium intake seem to correlate closely, inasmuch as nutritional needs are met with a diet based on protein, dairy products and legumes.

It is useful to underline that the intake of dairy products offers benefits for bone metabolism without leading to any increase in body weight, and least of all obesity in post-menopausal women who have a normal body weight[99]. A diet based on cheeses increases HDL cholesterol and reduces LDL cholesterol more than a diet dominated by meat or carbohydrates, and is inversely associated with cardiovascular risk. However, it must not be forgotten that cheese contains high percentages of sodium, which can raise the values of blood pressure.

Replacing animal fats with vegetable fats has a negative impact on bone and on muscle mass, but reduces the risk of all cardiac illnesses, such as a heart attack, heart failure, and stroke, with results that become appreciable after two years of sticking to this regime; they obtain benefits thereby for prevention in healthy individuals, and also as secondary prevention in persons who already have a critical cardiac condition[100].

Women who are overweight in post-menopause are more at risk than other women of the same age with normal body weight

---

99 Rautiainen, Wang, Lee *et alii*, *Dairy consumption in association with weight change and risk of becoming overweight or obese in middle-aged older women: A prospective cohort study*, in "Am J Clin Nutr", vol. 103, 2016 pp. 979–988.

100 Hopper, Summerbell, Thompson, *Reduced or modified dietary fat for preventing cardiovascular disease*, in "Cochrane Database of Systematic Reviews", vol. 6, 2011.

as regards all conditions that have a metabolic basis, and it is vital that they adopt the dietary regime most suited to their medical history, with the help of their attending doctor.

Risk of falls, and physical exercise

An important problem for elderly people is the risk of falling over, which can lead to damage to the joints and to the skeleton, with serious consequences, even when they are not particularly traumatic. Falls are frequent owing to the weakness of the muscles, the fact there is less firmness in the step, and unstable balance. Obviously, there are many individual variables, but a decline in walking ability has to be reckoned with for every person who reaches an advanced age.

Broken bones are harder to resolve than dislocated joints, and can condemn a person who is already frail to reduced mobility, with a resultant overall decline in the quality of life. Having freedom of movement means going outside, retaining the possibility of meeting people and cultivating interests, such as going to see shows, dining together with others, going to a recreational club, and so on. A motor impairment rarely allows a satisfying lifestyle, and instead condemns one to isolation.

Falls can be prevented by maintaining the funcionality of the limbs; this concept goes beyond the concept of mere bone health, because it involves the ability to maintain balance in posture. Training routines to improve body function that include exercises to strengthen the muscles, and to improve balance and walking skills, seem the ones most suited to this purpose, as long as they are carried out on a regular basis, at least three times a week. A preventive program is vitally important, considering that people over the age of 65 have a fall at least once a year, and that some of these falls may be traumatic.

Healthy women in post-menopause who engage in physical activity improve muscle strength and balance with undoubted benefits, although it is not possible to determine the percentage of falls that they manage to avoid compared to other, sedentary women of the same age[101]. The advantages of physical exercise are beyond question, especially post-menopause, when women lose the protective advantage of estrogens, and the tendency to be sedentary increases. Keeping one's weight under control reduces the frequency of diabetes, hypertension, hypercholesterolemia and heart disease, but it does not help to prevent traumas; physical exercise combats cognitive decline, mood swings, cardiovascular resistance and osteoporosis, and also increases muscle strength, flexibility and balance, with a total absence of contraindications or side effects.

---

101 McNamara, Gunter, *The influence of participation in Better Bones and Balance on skeletal health: Evaluation of a community-based exercise program to reduce fall and fracture risk*, in "Osteoporos Int", vol. 23, 2012, pp. 1813–1822.

Men, The Other Half of the Universe

Male sexual response with aging

Men do not experience an event similar to female menopause, but they do undergo the same kind of biological evolution that leads to aging in every living being. This process manifests itself with alterations affecting the vascular, endocrine, and neurological systems, and that change sexual function even in the absence of a specific medical condition.

Frequency of intercourse slows down, and the probability of remaining active diminishes hand in hand with the advancing years; above the age of 65, only just over 50% of men maintain regular function, and about half of them have a problem. Most often this involves a difficulty in obtaining or maintaining an erection, or a loss of desire, or of sexual satisfaction. In this age range, dysfunctions have a chronic evolution, and 14% of patients take medications or supplements to improve their sexual capability. Naturally, poor health is often associated with a severe clinical pattern[102].

The vascular system

As a man grows older, he is often subject to metabolic disorders that most often relate to the regulation of glycemia and blood pressure. Diabetes and hypertension are associated with

---

102 Lindau S.T., Schumm L.P., Laoumann E.O. *et alii, A study of sexuality and health among older adults in the United States*, in "N Engl J Med" vol. 357, 2007, pp. 762–774.

an inflammatory state of the vascular system, and effect erectile capability even when they are only moderate. Erectile dysfunction (ED) affects 5–20% of males, with symptoms varying from mild to severe. As it is a predominantly vascular pathology, ED is often associated with cardiovascular conditions (CVD), with which it shares risk factors such as a sedentary lifestyle and obesity; this is why it affects up to 70–95% of obese men[103]. The common ground upon which both cardiovascular disease and erectile dysfunction develop seems to be a pathology of the endothelium, meaning the lining of arteries and corpora cavernosa (the organs involved in an erection). The pathology is responsible for a reduction of blood flow into the corpora cavernosa, and consequently results in only a partial erection. The relationship between CVD and ED is so direct that the presence of a persistent erectile dysfunction must be considered an indication for coronary damage that has not yet become evident[104].

The endocrine system

The hypothalamic–pituitary–gonadal axis connects the central nervous system (CNS) and the gonads to regulate two functions that are essential for fertility: the production of sperm, and of the androgen hormones (male). The hypothalamic–pituitary–gonadal axis remains active throughout life, but it gradually slows down because of aging. With age, the volume of ejaculate, and the morphology, motility, and amount of spermatazoa diminish, making a man progressively less fertile. A statistically significant

103 Maiorino M.I., Bellastella G., Giugliano D. *et alii, From inflammation to sexual dysfunctions: A journey through diabetes, obesity, and metabolic syndrome,* in "Journal of Endocrinological Investigation", 2010, pp. 1–10.

104 Jackson G., Nehra A., Miner M. *et alii, The assessment of vascular risk in men with erectile dysfunction: The role of the cardiologist and general physician,* in "Int J Clin Pract", vol. 67, 2013, pp. 1163–1172.

inverse relationship has been observed between sperm quality and the patient's age, with the most significant alterations of the ejaculate being seen after age 55. Testosterone (T) loses its circadian rhythm, and is released irregularly because of the alterations in the endocrine balance that are specific to aging, and also because of collateral pathologies that are more frequent in older age. Indeed, other organs such as the liver and kidneys take part in hormonal regulation. Circulating T values diminish in the presence of liver cirrhosis, at levels that correlate with the severity of the condition; also a condition of chronic renal insufficiency reduces T levels, which, together with the vasculopathy and neuropathy characteristic of the pathology, lead to erectile difficulty.

Hypogonadism

Testosterone (T) is the pre-eminent male homone secreted by the gonads throughout a man's lifespan. Pathologies affecting the testicles (primary hypogonadism) and the pituitary (secondary hyopogonadism) alter the amount of testosterone production, and, consequently, the function of the biochemical processes that are regulated by the hormone. Both hypogonadisms recognize congenital, traumatic, tumoral, or iatrogenic causes, like radiation therapy.

Many chronic conditions that are associated with low circulating levels of T do not match the definition of primary or secondary hypogonadism given above. These conditions present themselves in adult age, and are characterized by a functional alteration of the pituitary and the testicles, without apparent cause. The syndrome of hypogonadism acquired in adult age (adult onset hypogonadism – AOH) has been defined recently; its relationship to the hypothalamus-pituitary-gonadal axis and its prevalence are not yet clear because, with aging, many men maintain adequate funtion, while many others develop a pattern of AOH.

The clinical pattern that follows the decrease of circulating testosterone is characterized by an absence of spontaneous night-time erections, and a loss of sexual desire and sexual ability, in addition to non-sexual symptoms such as mood swings, low energy, and deterioration in the subjective perception of well-being. Changes in metabolism and musculoskeletal function, an increase in body mass index, abdominal obesity, and metabolic syndrome are also conditions that characterize AOH, and that are associated with decreased testosterone production. Some medications (eg opioid analgesics, glucocorticoids, inhibitors of gastric secretion, and older kinds of antidepressants) contribute toward lowering testosterone, with alterations in a man's sleep architecture, sleep apnea, and psychosocial stress. Moreover, men who take high quantities of anabolizers may undergo a drastic reduction of T levels when the medication is discontinued. The clinical pattern becomes established only subtly, and progresses slowly, with muscle weakness, depression, and difficulty in concentrating that are difficult to define. A sexual dysfunction is often the first problem the patient actually notices.

AOH responds to lifestyle changes that promote physical activity and controlled nutrition. Weight loss, however it is obtained, increases T levels favorably. T supplementation (TRT) has positive effects on various parameters, but it has to be given for an extended period of time by experienced physicians, and the improvements obtained on sexual function and quality of life must be evaluated over the course of two or three years[105]. Prescribing T enhances well-being, parameters of sexual behavior, and somatic symptoms; at the same time, it ameliorates the response to oral medications for erectile dysfunction[106].

105 Khera M., Broderick G.A., Carson C.C. *et alii, Adult-onset hypogonadism*, in "Mayo Clin Proc", vol. 91, 2016, pp. 908–926.
106 Rosen R.C., Wu F., Behre H.M. et alii, *Quality of life and sexual function benefits effects of long-term testosterone treatment: Longitudinal results from the Registry of Hypogonadism in Men (RHYME)*, in "J Sex Med.", vol 14, 2017, pp. 1104–1115.

The neurological system

An alteration in peripheral neurological function affecting the lower limbs is common in people over 60, and its severity increases in line with age. This neurological deficit results in a difficulty in walking, keeping one's balance, and an increasing tendency to fall over, as well as pain and loss of sensitivity in the lower limbs that contributes further to reducing one's physical activity. This vicious circle further deteriorates one's neurological status. The direct link between difficulty of movement and reduced physical activity maintains this pathology, but also represents a "modifiable condition", meaning that it responds and gets better if the patient follows a specific physical rehabilitation program; laboratory tests confirm, indisputably, that physical activity is associated with better function, both motor and sensory, of the lower limbs.

Of the most common illnesses of older age, diabetes, characterized by peripheral neuropathy and vasculopathy, attacks both components of erection, and significantly alters the erotic response. Sexual problems that are secondary to diabetic neuropathy include erectile difficulty and retrograde ejaculation, which affect around 36% of these patients, three times as many as in the general population[107].

Prevention through nutrition

Wrong nutrition habits and a sedentary lifestyle are recognised as the prime causes of metabolic syndrome and of obesity, that are directly linked to hypogonadism and erectile dysfunction in the male. The good news is that when patients undertake a

---

107 Fedele D., *Therapy insight: sexual and bladder dysfunction associated with diabetes mellitus*, in "Nature clinical practice urology", vol. 2, 2005, pp. 282–290.

low-calorie regimen and lose weight, there is a clear increase in testosterone and in its carrier protein (SHBG), with improvement of erectile function. Risk factors for a metabolic condition, primarily cardiovascular disease, are thought to be modifiable, because every patient can change his or her eating habits and lifestyle, improving health expectations. Change is the most powerful weapon against predisposing factors, and the only way to prevention. Sooner or later, eating choices that favor the consumption of refined sugar and fat, and neglect fruit, vegetables, and fibers mean that one ends up being overweight or obese, precipitating a series of events that worsen the overall metabolic function. Getting stuck in wrong habits makes it more and more difficult to break down this vicious circle in favor of a healthier behavior. Specifically, to preserve endothelial function, which plays a crucial role in the male sexual response, a diet that favors fish and raw vegetables seems particularly indicated, while physical exercise must not be overlooked to improve global functioning[108].

The most common metabolic diseases, diabetes, hypertension, and cardiovascular problems have chronic patterns, and it is not likely that they will heal. They will rather worsen, or slowly reach a positive evolution thanks to an effective combination of treatment, eating regimen, and physical exercise. This is where the patient's ability to adapt his lifestyle to his health needs, and to maintaining a gratifying sexuality, comes into play.

---

108 van Bussel B.C., Henry R.M., Ferreira I. et alii, *A healthy diet is associated with less endothelial dysfunction and less low-grade inflammation over a 7-year period in adults at risk of cardiovascular disease*, in "J Nutr.", vol. 145, 2015, 532–540.

Aging mechanisms, orgasm, and sexuality in relationships

Despite the fact that popular wisdom says otherwise, both women and men retain an interest in sex throughout their lives, although it very much depends on personal situations like having a stable partner and on one's health status. For well-bonded couples, their sex life continues to represent a source of intimacy and pleasure, even in advanced age, in spite of inevitable physical problems. These mainly consist in vaginal atrophy in the case of women, and erectile difficulty for men. It is "curious" that the two pathologies have the same origin, ie the reduction of blood flow to the genitals, or, to be more precise, the inability to increase blood flow in response to sexual excitement. Vive la difference! We are more alike than we may think.

During erotic excitement, the genitals undergo the anatomical transformations that we all know, and that unfortunately are weakened by the mechanisms of aging: blood vessels and nerves in the genitals respond slowly, and require more powerful and lengthier stimulation to provide a good enough response. This prospect leads to resistance in many, while personal motivation and mutual support are key to overcoming the uncertainties, and finding effective stimuli.

In theory, lengthy manual stimulation should be welcomed, as it produces erotic pleasure, but often this is not the case. A woman is ashamed for needing so much time, she feels inadequate and is afraid that her partner will get bored. These intrusive thoughts interfere with the pleasurable sensations and make it harder and harder to get excited and to lubricate. The emotional distress triggers a mounting spiral of anxiety and negative expectations that is difficult to break down without the partner's support, and maybe some professional help. For his part, the man is not always ready to help his partner with prolonged stimulation, as he is also in a state of fragility, with erections that become weaker and weaker due to the effects of aging. Devoting so much time to her often means losing his own erection, and not being able to get it back for a certain amount of time. A man needs help from his partner, too, but becoming less ready to perform in an erotic context makes him feel inadequate and reluctant to ask for the kind of stimulation that would be welcome in any other circumstance.

Unfortunately, it is not easy to change. Many do not realize why what has always worked is not working now, and do not consider exploring new ways to improve their capability; other couples lack the motivation as, although harmonious in daily life, they cannot talk about sex, and so they don't even bother.

In general, a middle-aged couple's attitude is to value sexuality as long as it remains good without too much effort. When it becomes necessary to make an effort to understand what is no longer working, knowing that things will never be the same, many are ready to give up sex that has lost importance, rather than jeopardize the stability of the relationship. For that matter, as long as the partners share the same attitude, harmony is not in jeopardy. Conflicts arise when the couple wants different things: one would like an effort to be made to reinvent him- or herself, while the other prefers other aspects in the relationship. Often the two partners do not realize they have different expectations until a conflict arises; in these circumstances, sex therapy sessions provide the opportunity to express oneself and to listen to the other, helping the couple to meet each other halfway.

Further reading:

Kaplan H.S., *Sex, intimacy, and the aging process*, in "J. Am. Ac. Psychoanalysis", vol. 18, 1990.

Conclusions

Since the Second World War, technological developments in Western countries have seen an increase that is not comparable to those seen in any previous era, both in terms of the quantity of resources that were created and in terms of the speed with which the new "discoveries", or rather technical acquisitions, entered daily use.

A healthy home, drinking water, and education have changed people's health and awareness. In the medical field, not only are we able to treat conditions that were once incurable, we can even give early diagnoses or prescribe preventively, preventing a disease or illness from becoming established.

Study and exposure to information help to develop the awareness needed to make the best use of scientific reources; this is the scenario in which women live who today enter menopause: active 50-somethings who are educated and aware that they can benefit from knowledge and resources to carry out advance prevention against avoidable illnesses that this new physical state, as we have seen in the pages of this book, brings with it. In previous decades, the biochemistry of menopause was no different, nor was the attitude of women themselves (they were in control of their own lives back then, too); what has changed, rather, are the available resources, and this opens up a world of opportunities that did not exist for our grandmothers and great-grandmothers.

Menopause, with its repercussions on health and on the psycho-relational sphere, is a personal matter that each woman tends to manage privately, going to her doctor only for questions that seem to have clearly pathological implications.

This attitude is rather restrictive, because there are many issues which they could seek advice on, issues not necessarily strictly relating to actual health problems as such. Understanding how the metabolism evolves becomes an invitation to change one's behavior, preferring a healthy diet and physical exercise, in order to improve well-being.

Since many medical conditions are a result of incorrect nutrition, stressing the importance of nutrition and movement for maintaining a good quality of life as one grows older will never be wasted effort. Unfortunately, good intentions vanish and good habits do not last long after one or two counseling sessions; with a view to this, a source of information that remains available, and which one may turn to at various different times, helps to recognise the evolution of various psycho-physical aspects, and promises longer-lasting results.

The society we live in is not perfect, and the road to scientific knowledge will never end, but, at the same time, each person has a personal responsibility to work on their own internal growth, to make the best use of resources, and to accept what biology imposes.

Human beings are made up of *a body*, a machine with many organs that work, and fall ill, in synergy, and of *a psyche* made up of thoughts, feelings and emotions, the essential things that are not visible to the eye. The body and the mind are connected so closely that some medical conditions represent the individual's response to a psychical disturbance and, by the same token, an emotional attitude derives from a physical condition. The fact that anxiety leads to gastritis or insomnia, and that an invalidating or potentially fatal condition leads to depression are examples known to everyone, just as it is well-known that the physical ailments typical of menopause lead to emotional difficulty.

It should be stressed that the emotional reaction may be hidden by the appearance of a difficulty in the sexual sphere, which the patient does not see the reasons for, and which she does not connect with the state of menopause. The fact is that there is a link between problems with one's mood and sexual dysfunction, and it is well-known to those who study this subject; however, there is no point in this information remaining in the hands of the privileged few! Only if it is made more widely available can it reach people who are suffering and become a means of making things better. From the issues addressed herein, a person learns to recognise the link between the body, the psyche and sexuality, and can ask for help. Indeed, having a broad base of information available allows people to find the answer to their queries, and allows this resource to be used again and again, at several different times, increasing the chances of it being a valid means for prevention.

Being aware of the origin of a difficulty is the first step in resolving it, and if this book has helped to improve someone's knowledge, and stimulated their determination to ask for help, then it has achieved its purpose. It will then be up to the experts in the field to offer the best course of treatment for the individual case.

In writing this book, I have tried to present the event known as menopause in terms of its biological normality, and also to underline the pathological imperfections that most frequently occur on top of the particular physiological ailment, and that can become an illness.

My final recommendation is to accept with a certain lightness a situation that is unpleasant, and to use the preventive tools carefully. I would not have been able to say anything had many women not confided their problems in me, and for this reason I thank them.

No man is an island... and no woman is an island, either.

This book would not have existed without the benefit of the colleagues with whom I have built my professional training, and the medical school library services that have allowed me to continue to study. Many people have contributed to my professional training, which I regard as an ongoing process.

I wish to thank my mentors Helen S. Kaplan and William A. Frosch at the Cornell University Medical Center, New York City, and Raul C. Schiavi from the Mount Sinai Medical School, New York City, who, in differing ways, but in equally significant ways, have contributed to my professional growth. The manuscript was read by my friends Alessandra & Brunella, Antonella,

Helga, Letizia and Lucia, who gave me their encouragement and their affection.

There are two people who have made the biggest contribution to the drafting of this book: Dr Paolo Toti, a long-standing friend, who took it upon himself to read the early drafts, giving me specific and valuable advice for correcting and fine-tuning the imperfect medical information. The second is Mrs. LS, from the Bennici & Sirianni literary agency, who drew up the sequence of chapters and issues to be dealt with, helping me to organize my thoughts and my notes. Indeed, she gave me the narrative structure that I would not otherwise have been able to find by myself.

Finally, a word of thanks not to one person but to a whole institute: the Cornell University Medical Center, New York Presbyterian Hospital. Studying at Cornell made me a more creative person, and increased my confidence in myself.

To all these people, thank you!

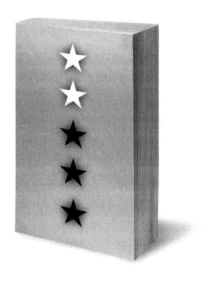

HERZ FÜR AUTOREN A HEART FOR AUTHORS À L'ÉCOUTE DES AUTEURS MIA KAPΔIA ΓIA ΣYΓΓP
RTA FOR FÖRFATTARE UN CORAZÓN POR LOS AUTORES YAZARLARIMIZA GÖNÜL VERELIM SZÍ
PER AUTORI ET HJERTE FOR FORFATTERE EEN HART VOOR SCHRIJVERS TEMOS OS AUTO
ZÖINKÉRT SERCE DLA AUTORÓW EIN HERZ FÜR AUTOREN A HEART FOR AUTHORS À L'ÉCOU
ÃO ВСЕЙ ДУШОЙ К АВТОРАМ ETT HJÄRTA FÖR FÖRFATTARE À LA ESCUCHA DE LOS AUTOI
EURS MIA KAPΔIA ΓIA ΣYΓΓPAФEIΣ UN CUORE PER AUTORI ET HJERTE FOR FORFATTERE EEN H
ARLARIMIZ   R   ZÖINKÉRT SERCE DLA AUTORÓW EIN HERZ FÜI
SCHRIJ   S O   ÇÃO ВСЕЙ ДУШОЙ К АВТОРАМ ETT HJÄRTA FÖI

The author

Born in the Medieval heart of Tuscany, Anna
Ghizzani moved to Florence to attend high school
and became fascinated with the art of Renaissance.
Graduating in modern languages shaped her
interest in history and cultures. Fascinated by
scientific thinking she attended medical school
developing an interest in reproduction and
prevention. This why she became an Ob/Gyn. After
residency, she got involved in the medical aspects
of sexuality, which brought her to attend the Sex
Therapy Program at Cornell Medical Center and
the Human Sexuality Program at Mt. Sinai Hospital,
in NYC. Clinical work, research and teaching at the
State Medical School in Siena have often combined
Sexual Medicine and Ob/Gyn expertise, focusing
on health issues and sexual dysfunctions for men
and women. Her main professional interest is in
the field of sexuality for men and women, couples'
issues, sexual pain, disorders of the lower genital
tract and menopause.

The publisher

*He who stops
getting better
stops being good.*

This is the motto of novum publishing, and our focus
is on finding new manuscripts, publishing them and
offering long-term support to the authors.
Our publishing house was founded in 1997, and since
then it has become THE expert for new authors and
has won numerous awards.

**Our editorial team will peruse each manuscript
within a few weeks free of charge and without
obligation.**

You will find more information about
novum publishing and our books on the internet:

w w w . n o v u m p u b l i s h i n g . c o m